IRON HEART

IRON HEART

THE TRUE STORY OF HOW I CAME BACK FROM THE DEAD

Brian Boyle
with Bill Katovsky

Introduction by Gail McGovern,
President of the American Red Cross

SKYHORSE PUBLISHING

Skyhorse Publishing books may be purchased in bulk at special discounts for sales promotion, corporate gifts, fund-raising, or educational purposes. Special editions can also be created to specifications. For details, contact the Special Sales Department, Skyhorse Publishing, 307 West 36th Street, 11th Floor, New York, NY 10018 or info@skyhorsepublishing.com.

Skyhorse® and Skyhorse Publishing® are registered trademarks of Skyhorse Publishing, Inc.®, a Delaware corporation.

www.skyhorsepublishing.com

10 9 8 7 6 5

486 0249

Library of Congress Cataloging-in-Publication Data is available on file.
Hardcover ISBN: 978-1-60239-771-2
Paperback ISBN: 978-1-61608-360-1

Printed in the United States of America

As each second ticked by, my life was slipping away.

This book is dedicated to my mom and dad, the faculty and staff of Prince George's Hospital and the many others that have helped with my recovery.

You are the reason I am alive and breathing today.

Since 2007, I have worked very closely with the American Red Cross. It has been a true honor for me to volunteer, take part in their testimonial speaking engagements and blood drives, and to proudly wear their logo on my race suits during my triathlon and running events. I lost 60 percent of my blood at the scene of my accident, and Red Cross blood donors were there for me. As my treatment progressed, blood donors became a vital factor in my recovery and journey back into life.

Blood is needed for emergencies like mine, and for people undergoing treatment for cancer, those with chronic blood disorders, premature babies, people in need of surgery, and many others. For the nearly 5 million people who receive blood transfusions every year, your blood donation can make the difference between life and death. I am living proof of this.

When I needed it, the American Red Cross was there with 36 blood transfusions and 13 plasma treatments that saved my life in a situation where time was of the essence. Volunteer blood donors made this possible. By giving just a little bit of their time, blood donors gave me a lifetime.

On behalf of the many patients like me to whom you have given a second chance, a heartfelt thank you to all Red Cross blood donors.

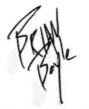

CONTENTS

Part Two: Body

Part Three: Soul

INTRODUCTION

As president and CEO of the American Red Cross, I have the great privilege of meeting ordinary people who have done extraordinary things in times of disaster and emergency—individuals who rush in to help when everyone else is running away.

Each year our employees and volunteers respond to seventy thousand disasters, in communities small and large. In addition to responding to disasters, the American Red Cross trains ten million people each year in everything from first aid and CPR to aquatics and babysitting. Travelling across the country visiting local Red Cross chapters, I have had the honor of recognizing many individuals who have put these skills to use, saving the life of a family member, neighbor, or even a complete stranger. In Indianapolis, I met a fourteen-year-old and her grandparents who, together, pulled a four-year-old child out of a lake after she had fallen through the ice. They performed CPR for eight minutes, and the child is miraculously alive and well. I've honored a young boy for performing the Heimlich maneuver on his choking three-year-old brother. And even at our national headquarters, an employee recently saved the life of another who had gone into cardiac arrest by performing CPR until an ambulance arrived. There are countless stories, but I never cease to be amazed by the courage, action, and selflessness of those I meet through the Red Cross.

But I've never encountered a more inspiring story or individual than Brian Boyle. He is anything but ordinary—he is a miracle. And he is a hero.

Brian was actually the recipient of an American Red Cross service—blood. The American Red Cross is the largest single supplier of blood and blood products in the United States, collecting and processing more than forty percent of the blood supply and distributing it to some three thousand hospitals and transfusion centers nationwide. This adds up to ten million units of blood each year. Every two seconds someone receives a unit of blood, and we are grateful to the many individuals who take an hour of their day to roll up their sleeve and donate this precious gift of life.

As you will read in this incredible account, Brian lost *sixty* percent of his blood after a nearly fatal car accident at the age of eighteen. In addition to fouteen lifesaving surgeries, Brian had thirty-six blood transfusions and thirteen plasma treatments. After two months in the ICU fighting for his life, Brian made a miraculous recovery. Brian did more than just recover, however—he was reborn. Three years after his accident, Brian completed the 2007 Ironman World Championship in Hawaii and has been a competitive athlete ever since. He also became a beloved spokesperson for the American Red Cross.

We're extremely proud and honored to have Brian representing the American Red Cross. Brian makes an incredible impact as he shares his powerful story and reminds countless individuals of the need to give blood. For every individual he encourages to donate blood, he is helping to save up to three lives. He visits high schools and colleges to promote blood drives and will soon be embarking on a national campaign for the Red Cross. As Brian continues to compete in triathlons and marathons, he also proudly wears the American Red Cross logo as a tribute to the blood donors that helped to save his life. He was awarded the American Red Cross Regional Spokesperson of the Year award in 2009 and 2010. And last year, he also made his very first blood donation at the hospital that brought him back to life.

Each time I speak with Brian, he thanks me profusely for what I do for the Red Cross, when, in fact, Brian is the one who cannot be thanked enough. I am in awe of Brian's physical stamina, sheer determination, and his accomplishments as an Ironman athlete. But most of all, I'm in awe of Brian's tenacity, relentless energy, graciousness, dedicated spirit, and compassionate commitment to helping others. I'm convinced that he is superhuman.

In the summer of 2004, thirty-six generous individuals took one hour out of their day to donate blood. These thirty-six individuals gave Brian a second at chance at life. We are extraordinarily grateful to each and every one of our blood donors. There is no gift as precious as the gift of life, and no one acknowledges this more than Brian Boyle. Brian treats each day as a gift and an opportunity to help others. I know that after reading Brian's remarkable journey of courage and determination, you will be as moved and inspired by him as I continue to be.

Gail McGovern,
President of the American Red Cross

PART ONE

HEART

CHAPTER 1

WAKING UP

I AWAKE TO REGULAR BEEPING SOUNDS. I'M ALONE IN A WHITE ROOM AND looking straight up at the ceiling. Bright lights shine all around me. My heart is beating fast. I try to raise my arms, then legs, but I can't move them. My head won't budge either. I can't blink or wiggle my fingers.

So what's making those pings and blips? It sounds like a machine, perhaps several. But what are they doing? One machine creates a small burst of air that gently caresses my face. Its slight breeze does not cool my hot skin. I feel beads of sweat pooling on my forehead. When the perspiration rolls down my cheeks and reaches my chapped lips, it soothes them because they are unbelievably dry. My throat is sore and irritated.

A figure dressed in all black appears. Could this be Death? I then notice a small white collar around his neck. Death looks like a priest. Do I know this man? Even so, I can't recognize him because his face remains a blur. Suddenly, my mind swells with a screaming sound. It's a loud, almost deafening noise, as if the priest is yelling in my ear. The sound vibrations are pounding inside my skull, like I'm standing in front of giant speakers at a rock concert. Then the noise somehow turns into actual words spoken in a slow, distorted tone. I strain to make sense of his words: "In the name of the Father and of the Son and of the Holy Spirit . . . " Why is he giving me the last rites? I try to shut down my brain so his words won't affect me. I want him to stop or go away. The room goes dark.

I'M AWAKE. THE PRIEST IS GONE. EVERYTHING IN MY BODY FEELS NUMB. I want to close my eyes, but they won't move or shut. I feel tears welling up. It's like I'm underwater looking up at the surface. With this sensation, a vivid memory arises. I'm suddenly back at the outdoor pool where I used to swim with my younger cousins Matt and Hayley.

"Hey, Matt, watch this!" It has just started to rain and I dive into the water. Through my swim goggles I peer upward at the gray sky, trying to see anything above the water past the reflection and through the many raindrops colliding with the surface. I feel weightless and at peace underwater.

But I'm not in a pool right now. My attention returns to my burning eyes. They feel like they've been open for hours, maybe even days. Is that even possible? Wouldn't they dry out at some point? This thought makes me nauseous; I want to vomit, but that urge is overwhelmed by something even more powerful. My left arm feels like it's on fire. The pain is excruciating. *Somebody throw water on me. Please! I'm begging you!*

No one comes because I can't speak. So I suffer in isolation and maddening silence. My mind goes blank. I can't remember anything, not even my name. Somehow, without urgent prompting, I remember: *Yes, my name is Brian. Brian Boyle. Am I dead?* But if I were dead, I wouldn't be able to have these thoughts because dead people can't think, right? But I don't feel normal or alive either. Something is terribly wrong.

Maybe this is just a bad dream. So let's try something to wake up. I can bite my tongue. Bite. Bite and wake up. But I can't bite my tongue because I can't even feel it. Where is it? It has to be in my mouth somewhere. I try again. If I had a tongue in this nightmare it would probably have been bitten off by now. I bite harder. Nothing.

My heart starts beating faster. Its thumping rhythm rises above the eerie silence that's filled my mind. But why is it beating in the center of my chest, which isn't where the heart is located? And something heavy must be sitting on my chest because it's crushing me. The pressure increases. I want to shout, "Get this thing off me, I can't breathe," but I can't make a sound. My heart feels like it's going to explode.

An alarm starts beeping loudly. I see red lights flashing. This is real; it's not happening in a dream.

I hear footsteps. Several. Now I feel many hands on me. Grabbing my feet, arms, head. The hands pick me up, and I'm placed on a table with wheels. *Why? What are you doing? And where are you taking me?*

Blurry shadows of people cluster around me. Voices are talking loud and fast: something about my heart and emergency surgery. Does this mean that I'm in a hospital? And what's wrong with my heart? Oh man, this can't be good. *Mom, Dad, where are you? I need you.*

I'm being pushed down all these different hallways. The ceiling looks the same everywhere—large white rectangular sheets of tile broken up by fluorescent lights with clear plastic covers.

The gurney is moving quickly, with several people running alongside. They're also dragging the beeping machines. A large man looms over me. Underneath his white lab coat, he's wearing a light blue button-up shirt. There's a ballpoint pen and two red markers in his front pocket. He's wearing an identification card connected to a lanyard. I struggle to read the name: DR. JAMES CATEVENIS, ICU DIRECTOR, PRINCE GEORGE'S HOSPITAL CENTER.

ICU. That's . . . Intensive Care Unit! This has gone from bad to worse. Only people who are critically injured or near death find themselves in Intensive Care.

The moving bed slams into a set of folding doors that swing open. I'm being wheeled into a partially lit room. It's quiet here. Voices echo off the aqua-green tile walls. The bed comes to a complete stop and many hands surround me again, lifting my body onto a cold, hard surface.

People huddle near me. Everyone is wearing light blue surgical wardrobes and white latex gloves. A wide overhead light flicks on; it's bright as the sun. Someone squirts brownish liquid on my chest and rubs it in, and another person places a clear plastic mask over my nose and mouth. A cool, scentless breeze fills the mask.

I stare up at one of the doctors who stands to my left. He must be the head surgeon because he's directing everyone. He says something about fluid building up around my heart. I watch his hands hover near my chest. He's holding a shiny object, which looks sharp, like a scalpel. The overhead light grows brighter. Within seconds, it swallows me in an even brighter flash. The last thing I hear before losing consciousness is the surgeon: "Let's hope the third time is the charm."

CHAPTER 2

HOPING TO FIND ANSWERS AND FINDING NONE

I'M IN A NEW ROOM. I HEAR FOOTSTEPS, THEN THE SOUND OF SHUFFLING papers. A machine starts up in front of me—the rumble of an air conditioner combined with a microwave's hum. Some footsteps come closer. My bed shakes and moves, but only for a few feet, then halts. The ceiling looks different. I must be near a wall because I see dark areas that could be pictures or posters. My eyes are frozen, staring straight ahead. I can't quite see what the posters are, so I try to move my head but I can't. I see the letter *R* on one of them, in my peripheral vision. The word is a long one, whatever it is. Maybe I'll be able to see it if my bed starts to move again.

The faint scent of flowers, maybe perfume, pleases me. I see the shadow of a woman standing nearby. A nurse? I wish she would say something.

Papers rustle. The scent of perfume is stronger now. She speaks in a soft whisper: "Brian Boyle, eighteen years old, motor vehicle accident victim, ICU patient since July 6, 2004."

Motor vehicle accident? July 6? I don't remember a thing. No memory of it, just an empty space.

"Brian, can you hear me?" she says loudly into my right ear, startling me. "If you can hear me, blink your eyes. No? Okay, can you squeeze my hand?" She grabs my right hand. "Come on, I know you can do it, buddy. Squeeze my hand just a little bit." She gives it a subtle squeeze but she gets no response in return—no movement whatsoever. "We are all waiting for you to get better. Just hang in there."

Hang in there? Where else can I go? But why do I keep having these weird feelings in the middle of my chest? I feel my heart's regular beating—*thump, thump, thump*.

"Okay, Mr. Boyle, you're next in line for a CAT scan. Same procedure as this morning. You should be used to it by now." As she walks away, I hear her mutter under her breath, "Poor kid, he's already been through so much."

My mind explodes into a thousand fragments. I see myself walking through a minefield. The ground is made of golden yellow sand, and every few steps that I take, I accidentally set off one of the mines. *Boom.* There go my legs. My body falls to the ground, but I carry on in shock, dragging forward what's left of me. I set off another mine with my hand. *Boom.* There goes my left arm. I'm on my back now, bleeding to death, trying to pull myself through the sand with my right arm. I struggle to move a few inches, all the while begging God for answers. I look up at the blue sky, miserable, searching for one last bit of hope. My eyes are burning from the sun's brightness. I then see a small dot in the cloud. Salvation? The dot is getting bigger. The dot becomes this date—July 6.

But what day is it now? And why did she say that I'm used to this? How many of these CAT scans have I had? And just exactly what is a CAT scan? *Hey, Ms. Nurse, come back and tell me more!*

Those papers she was looking at are right behind me. They must be attached to my bed or something. If I could grab them, I'd get some answers. I try to lift my left arm. Nothing. I try harder. Nothing! Why is this so difficult? What about my other arm? It won't move, either.

My body feels warm. Cool drops of sweat pool on my forehead, slowly pausing at my eyebrows. But when the sweat rolls into my eyes, it burns like acid. I can't do anything to stop the pain, but at least I feel pain. I stare at the ceiling, trying to think of something else.

What is that word on the side of the wall, the one that starts with the *R*? It's driving me batty. Maybe if I can figure out what that word is, I can start figuring out why I'm here.

I shift my attention to the ceiling, then the wall, then back to the ceiling. I count the little specks of holes in the ceiling. My throat is dry; I desperately need water.

My mind returns to the unexplained, totally baffling reality of being in Intensive Care. I hear footsteps again. They are coming from behind, off to the right. It must be the woman. I smell her perfume. She is close, fidgeting with some machine. I hear the click and clack of buttons being pressed. Am I about to enter the CAT scan machine? I don't know why, but I feel like I'm about to enter the slaughterhouse.

An electronic beeping starts and I sense motion. I'm moving forward on some kind of conveyer belt and getting closer to the machine. It's a looming big white plastic mountain dotted with countless small neon green lights.

The machine stops. It's swallowed me whole and I'm its hostage. A frightening, cold robotic voice says: "Please hold your breath for thirty seconds." I try to obey the machine's stern command but can't hold my breath. My lungs are expanding and contracting on their own.

"Please hold your breath for thirty seconds," the voice repeats. *Hey, can you give me a moment?* I want to yell, *I can't do this! Take the damn scan already!* I try to hold my breath again, but can't. My heart and brain are racing to see which can go faster, and my heart takes the lead. The neon lights fade, the buzzing gets louder. Liquid fire returns to my left arm. I'm nauseous and dizzy.

The machine spits me back out. Perhaps it didn't like my taste.

I am naked. A soft breeze flows over me. My body is rigid, stiff as a plank of wood. The room is quiet, except for the beeping I heard when I was back in that other room. I drift off because my mind prefers to go on standby.

Then I hear a soft whisper from an elderly woman. "Hail Mary, full of grace, the Lord is with thee." My right hand is slightly raised, as if someone is holding it. "Blessed art thou among women, and blessed is the fruit of thy womb, Jesus." I can't see her because my eyes are taped shut. All I see is the gloomy, dark hue inside my eyelids. The voice continues, "Now and at the hour of our death." She begins reciting the rosary. Why is she saying this? And how did she know I'm Catholic? As she recites each line, darkness descends once more, like a welcoming friend offering me escape.

I emerge from what must be deep sleep. I'm not sure how long I have been out. I don't even know what to call it when everything goes dark and my mind turns off. Another day or two or three has passed; I can't tell. Fortunately, my eyelids are no longer taped closed. My vision is blurry, but I notice a large white space above me. Yes, the ceiling. It seems familiar. I'm back in the first room.

But why is my heart racing? I'm sweating profusely, or is it blood? Maybe both? I'm drenched in some disgusting broth and it feels like it's oozing out of my left side. I want to look down, but I can't move my head, though I have a peculiar prickly sensation running from head to toe. The pain is like a thousand needles stabbing me. My skin is getting hotter, and I feel at any moment my body will burst into flames. But at the same time, I am chilled, as if there are ice packs jammed under my arms and legs.

I still hear the fan's whirr. Every now and then, a small alarm goes off, and then a beeping begins. It seems like a nurse comes in every fifteen minutes. I can only guess, since time has no meaning. The nurses keep telling me that I've been in a serious car accident, but I have no recollection of an accident. The last thing I remember is my family's Fourth of July picnic held on July 3.

The picnic takes place every year and is organized by my dad's concrete construction company. My mom and I always tag along as my dad's guests, but even so, he spends most of the time reintroducing us to his coworkers. The day is warm and sunny. I smell hot dogs and hamburgers cooking on the grill. Kids are playing and laughing in the background. Layered over those sounds are several conversations taking place among the adults.

I step away from the crowd and walk toward a large grassy field. I want to get away from all the commotion and reflect on my plans for the fall. I'm looking forward to attending St. Mary's College of Maryland— which is only an hour away from home. In the spring of my high school senior year, my parents and I met with their swim coach, Andre Barbins.

I had a 4.0 grade point average, took several advanced placement courses, and was captain of my high school swim team, which was top-ranked in the state. Andre told me that I was going to be one of his top recruits. For the first few weeks of summer, I trained in the pool at the local recreation center while helping my dad with odd jobs like landscaping or going out to work sites with him.

I walk back to the crowded picnic and stay for the fireworks. That's the last thing I remember from the picnic, or anything else, before everything turns blank. My memory ceases from that point on.

I take a closer inspection of the room. The ceiling is etched in my brain; I've grown accustomed to its speckled pattern. One afternoon, when nurses are changing my gown and have turned me over, I see the room is crowded with at least a dozen electrical monitors.

A nurse enters my room. "Brian, honey, can you blink for me today?" she asks in a tone suggesting that she really isn't expecting an answer. I try to blink, but it's impossible. She gently rolls me on my right side while she checks a tube connected with the left part of my stomach. I now have a new view of the right side of the room that I haven't seen before. I realize that the fan is not a fan at all. I look closer at the small label that says Ventilator in big bold letters. I have a machine breathing for me. That's why I couldn't hold my breath in the CAT scan machine. If all these machines are keeping me alive, what does that mean? The white ceiling dims to charcoal.

CHAPTER 3

A NEW KIND OF LIVING HELL

ONE MORNING, THE SLIDING GLASS DOOR TO MY ROOM IS OPEN. My bed is raised at a slight incline, but my angle of view is limited since I can't move my head or eyes. Doctors and nurses are walking around in white coats and light blue scrubs. I recognize one whose face I saw on his identification card, Dr. James Catevenis. He checks on me frequently. He's drinking coffee, talking to a nurse who looks like she had a rough morning. Orderlies and nurses roll along people of all ages, some still connected to IVs, on gurneys.

A middle-aged woman and her daughter stop by my open door to ask a nurse a question. The daughter peeks into my room; then her eyes widen and she shouts, "Mommy, there's a monster in that room!" The woman glances at me and then says to her, "Oh, good Lord, honey, don't look at him." She grabs her daughter and rushes off. My mind sinks in absolute shame. I'm no longer human, just a half creature kept alive by machines like in a horror film. What have I done to deserve such harsh, unjust punishment?

An alarm goes off and everyone rushes to the room on my right. It blares for several minutes before ceasing. Soon, a gurney with a white sheet covering the body appears in the hallway. I'm starting to envy ICU patients en route to the morgue. At least their suffering is over and they are at peace. What if I have to spend the rest of my life trapped like this? Why should it be otherwise? I have all the time in the world to ponder this matter.

Every time a nurse or doctor enters my room, I can only stare at them like a wax figure. Motionless as a corpse, I can't talk, nod, lift a finger, or blink. When the doctors look right at me, they seem to be trying to read my mind. What I would give to have a simple conversation with these strangers. Instead, I'm lifeless, unmoving, unresponsive—a silent body trapped in a bed, with my arms spread out like a crucifixion on a mattress.

A nurse approaches holding a syringe. "Brian, you've been on a lot of really heavy medication, but we are going to try to wean your body off of all of that," she says. "We want you to get nice and healthy and strong. I'm going to just take some blood right now. Just a slight pinch and it will all be over."

The needle stings, and then she walks out of my room carrying a big bag of my blood. Several moments later, she returns and disappears behind my bed. Then, out of nowhere, vibrations start coming from under the bed, and I hear the pumping sound of hydraulics. My bed starts to move, reclining then rotating left. Am I going to slide off? I try to grab the sheets, but my stiff wooden fingers won't cooperate. With my body weight shifting, I feel pressure on my elbows, forehead, hips, and calves, wherever I'm strapped to the bed. The bed halts until I'm facing the wall at a ninety-degree angle. Blood rushes to my body's left side, causing an odd tingling sensation.

With this new view, I take in part of the room I've never seen before. It's all so foreign. I feel like a traveler arriving on a deserted island, exploring new exotic sights, sounds, and smells. I'm giddy. There are so many new things to examine.

The floor is made of shiny pinkish tiles with random specks of dark blue, purple, and brown colors. There's a wooden chair with an aqua-green cushion. I wonder how many people have sat in that chair over the years. Behind the chair is a tan-colored table with several drawers and a metal sink built into it. I'm not sure how big the sink is, but I can see the faucet and the container of soap next to it. I deeply crave a drink of water. The inside of my mouth is raw and dry as sandpaper. There are small white boxes on the left side of the sink containing bandages and latex gloves. The wall is an off-white color with a five-inch purple section in its middle. There's a white bulletin board with a card pinned next to it: Room 19Brian Boyle.

Okay, so I'm in Room 19. I still want to know what day it is and how I got in here in the first place. I want to know where my parents are and why I'm hooked up to these machines, and why my bed just rotated. Does anyone realize that I am not brain-dead? I want to scream!

For some reason, my body begins to shake. I can't control these tremors that begin to escalate in intensity. I'm shaking like a rag doll in a dog's mouth. As my teeth grind, my mouth foams up. I taste the awful metallic tang of blood, and feel the disgusting broth of bloodied saliva dripping down the left side of my face. I'm drifting in and out of consciousness; everything is hazy. Then everything calms down, although iron-tasting foam continues to leak from my mouth.

I'm exhausted, spent. My only thought is finding relief from this torture where I'm indifferently punished by a nameless, cruel force.

I'M STARING LISTLESSLY AT THE WALL. TIME PASSES. THEN SOMETHING bizarre happens. My eyes move! I don't know how this occurred, or if it was simply an assortment of neurons randomly and suddenly firing away deep inside the brain, but my eyes are finally able to slowly move within their sockets. They are no longer frozen.

The hydraulic system underneath the bed starts back up and I'm returned to the original flat position, but with a slight incline. While I still can't move my head, my eyeballs are free to roam, to take in more sights of the room. I don't know how long this visual freedom will last, so I hurry to take advantage of the new opportunity. I notice a clock above the door and small television set in the upper right corner of my room. After a while, my bed rotates back to the left.

Now I can see the bulletin board covered with photos. Many are of me from my high school graduation; others are from various swim meets. That's odd. Who put them there? There are also photos of my parents, relatives, and friends. Thinking of the life I used to have makes me sad. Tears well up around my lids and the salty liquid trickles down my cheeks, joining the trail of blood, foam, and saliva.

My body begins to tremble again, and then I'm violently shaking all over. I wait for the terrorizing frenzy to pass. After a minute or so, I'm finally released from its wicked grip. My pulse is rapid. What is wrong?

Suddenly, I blink! I try to blink again, but my eyelids feel heavy and restrained. I struggle to shut my eyes, and then try to reopen them. This takes awhile; I feel like a crane operator hoisting a steel beam with his eyelids. Finally, they are open. But relief is short-lived when I notice a treelike contraption by the bed—a nest of tubes, medical equipment, and containers filled with reddish liquid that's light in color and has a thick, slimy, gooey appearance. The mysterious stuff fills several plastic containers. A bright red tube comes out of the top of one these slime-filled containers, and interweaves with other wires and containers, then continues right down to the side of my body. Is this the medical brew keeping me alive? I look away in disgust. At that instant, a bubbling noise erupts from one of those containers and several teaspoons of liquid ooze into the tube, making a light gurgling noise.

CHAPTER 4

I RECOGNIZE MY PARENTS

I'm constantly thirsty. I can't remember the last time I had something to drink. My mouth is kept permanently open for a tube that goes down my throat, and some type of cool liquid is always dribbling down my chin. I can't even swallow; this is pathetic. How I yearn for a big glass of ice-cold water. My tongue feels like a shriveled-up piece of useless flesh. I thought the human body couldn't survive more than a few days without water. What's even worse is when the nurses and doctors wash their hands in the sink in my room. Listening to the water pour out from the small faucet, just a few feet away from my bed, is pure torment.

One day, a new nurse shows up. She is about five feet tall, short brown hair, thin, with a friendly disposition. She holds a clear plastic bottle and a yellow sponge. She walks up to me, not saying anything, and pours liquid from the bottle onto the sponge. I can't read the label but the liquid is clear. Wow, that's a strong odor. It smells like rubbing alcohol. She starts rubbing the damp sponge onto my legs, feet, arms, and the rest of my body. It tingles. I wonder what would happen if she gave me a swig of rubbing alcohol? This is how desperate my thirst is. When she leaves, my mind fixates on the out-of-reach sink.

I'M AWAKE. I DON'T KNOW HOW LONG I WAS OUT. WHAT I DREAD MOST are the terrifying dreams that can come at any time whenever I descend into what might loosely be called sleep. These dreams are unlike any I ever had during my old life. They're more vivid, with brighter colors and more extreme events. Could the medication be affecting my dreams? And exactly what medications are they?

Because I'm caught in a precarious limbo between life and death, it's not easy to detect what's real or a dream. They often swap places without warning, which only leaves me more anxious and baffled. What I would give to step outside my body for the briefest moment and look at the figure lying motionless in Room 19. Maybe I would find some answers.

I HAVE A DREAM THAT I AM SITTING UPRIGHT IN A CHAIR. I'M NO LONGER in the hospital room, but at the airport. Passengers are waiting to board and people are walking through the corridors as they exit the planes. The airport looks familiar. A sign says REAGAN NATIONAL AIRPORT. I have my portable CD player and I'm wearing headphones. I hear the smooth reggae rhythms of Bob Marley. I turn the volume up.

I'm wearing a damp white cotton T-shirt along with a pair of black mesh shorts with silver stripes. I reek of chlorine and my hair is wet. I bounce my Teva-clad right foot to the rhythm of the Jamaican music, but my heel is rubbing against something. I look down and notice a small black duffel bag under my chair. I guess I'm taking this with me onto the plane. Yet where am I going? Or have I already arrived and I'm waiting for someone? The next track on the CD is a good one. I love "Satisfy My Soul."

I pick up the bag and search its contents. There's a water bottle, wet black swimsuit, damp blue-striped towel, and a pair of goggles. Did I just come from swim practice? There is a feminine voice on the intercom that says one of the planes from American Airlines is boarding in twenty minutes. I don't have a ticket. I check the pockets in my shirt and look in my bag again, nothing. A hint of tension is building in my stomach because something doesn't feel right about this whole situation.

The lights throughout the airport concourse start to dim, and then shut off completely. Only sunlight illuminates the inside of the airport. An air-horn siren starts to go off, and I jump out of my seat and run to the exit, gripping my CD player.

Adrenaline pumping, I sprint around people, trying to reach a safer location. Wait! I forgot my bag. I have to go back and retrieve it. I find it, but pause. People are moving toward the exit. I can barely hear Marley, and now everything begins to move in slow motion. Then everything and everyone disappear. All I see is white. I'm now enclosed in a large white tube or some sort of bubble, and a strong blinding light is shining right at me. I don't know where I am, but I don't feel frightened; I sense that I'm not alone. I hear soft voices. An unfamiliar boy sits to my left, talking on a cell phone. He has short brown hair and is wearing a blue T-shirt. To my right are many boys and girls in chairs. It's almost like we are all gathered in a large waiting room, but what exactly are we waiting for? There must be hundreds of these young kids, and they all seem to be my age. The atmosphere is calm and relaxing.

The boy to my left with the phone asks if I need to use it or if he could call anyone for me. I tell him to call my parents. Seconds later, he reaches my parents and asks me what I would like him to say. I reply, "Could you tell my parents that I love them?"

Then I hear: "Brian, son, your mom and I want you to know that everything is going to be okay."

Dad? Could his voice not be part of my dream? Then where is he? I see a shadowy figure looming by my feet. I study his face. *Dad? Is that you? It is! You're here!* At long last! For the first time since my mind went blank, I see him in my room. I want to ask, "Where's Mom? Is she with you?" But I can't speak or blink or show any sign of communication to let him know that I recognize him. Excited, my pulse quickens and the machines start their pinging and beeping.

"Calm down son, it's okay," he says. He struggles to speak. Someone is standing behind him. *Mom?* I see her blonde hair. I can only shout to myself, *Mom, it's you! Oh, Mom, you're here! I'm so happy.* The beeping and buzzing machines get louder.

Two nurses flank my mom. They are holding her upright. She can barely look at me. Her face is hidden behind a veil of crumpled tissues that she holds in a trembling hand. In fact, her entire body is quivering. *Mom, don't be upset,* I want to say. Yet, I can only look at her with a frozen unblinking expression. She suddenly rushes out of the room.

My dad, however, stays at my side. I hear Bob Marley playing. That must be why I was hearing reggae in my dream. Dad starts gently rubbing my feet, massaging the toes as if they are made of glass. He's quiet, subdued, and looks like he has aged ten years since the July picnic. He barely maintains eye contact with me for more than a few seconds before glancing away. I watch a tear slide down his left cheek. He tells me that I'm in Prince George's Hospital, that I was in a bad car accident, that I have a few broken bones, and that I will be able to leave the hospital in several days. I sense that it's much worse than several broken bones, and his tense, pained look confirms my suspicion.

CHAPTER 5

ANGELS IN THE HALLWAY

THE NEXT TIME MY PARENTS VISIT, I WANT TO LET THEM KNOW THAT I'm right here. Their son might be buried inside the rigid shell of his unresponsive body, but his mind remains active, alert, internally engaged, though a bit dulled from the drugs or mysterious brown liquid pumped into his side. Yet how can I convey this, since I can't speak or even nod my head? My reality is this: I'm cut off from the world. Remove the life-support machines and I am dead.

Am I in what is known as a vegetative state? But surely this can't be the case; I'm aware of what is happening all around me. A cauliflower or artichoke doesn't ask itself what it's like to be picked in the field only to end up on someone's plate. But I'm scared that doctors and nurses seem to presume I'm a vegetable. "You used to be known as Brian Boyle, but that's all changed. Sorry buddy, but there's little difference between you and the leafy greens in the produce aisle."

I wait for my parents, still uncertain about what to do. As usual, my dad approaches the bed while my mom stands by the open door with two nurses. He says hi and begins to massage my feet. "Brian, can you move your feet?" he asks. "Come on son, wiggle your toes at least." I try to find some kind of sensation in my feet, but nothing. "Okay, well, how about blinking? Let's try that. Blink if you want me to keep rubbing your feet."

I stare at him, listening to the sad desperation in his voice. I have to blink. He needs this sign very much. I struggle to shut my eyes. It takes several seconds for the reflex to begin. With my eyes closed, I pause. A few moments later, I will myself to open my eyes. It's like I'm pushing a heavy boulder uphill with my eyelids. As soon as they open, he looks as if he has just witnessed a miracle. "Yes! You did it! I'm so proud of you!" he says. I blink again, this time in half as much time. It's getting easier. I continue to stare at him.

"JoAnne, watch this!" yells my dad. "You're not going to believe what Brian just did. He blinked!" My mom approaches my bed, looking more shell-shocked than curious.

My dad asks what I want to hear. He steps away, grabs a stack of my old CDs from a bag, and holds up *Led Zeppelin IV*. "Blink if you want me to play it," he says. "Mom is here. Show her that you can blink. Come on, son. You can do it."

I shut my eyes, pause for a second, and then launch my eyelids triumphantly. She gasps, putting her hand to her mouth in disbelief, and touches my right arm. Trembling and smiling, she keeps dabbing her reddened eyes with a tissue.

The song "Rock and Roll" plays softly in the background. I no longer hear the beeps and buzzes of the machines. Listening to Led Zeppelin with my parents, I no longer feel alone. My dad is sitting in the chair to my left, while my mom sits in the chair next to the wall on my right. They are both quiet. I suddenly feel movement in my feet. They are swaying several inches to the beat. My mom notices first. "Garth, look!" she cries. He sees my feet moving and rushes over to the foot of my bed.

"I can't believe it!" he shouts. He touches my feet to feel them moving as if seeing them shake isn't enough evidence. He tells me to stop moving them, and I do. Seeking an explanation, he turns around to the two nurses, who are standing just outside the sliding glass door. One says that the movement is possibly the result of a lower dosage of medication. My dad asks me to push my feet forward against his hands and I happily oblige. The two nurses hug each other with joy. The hallway lights silhouette them as if they are angels.

CHAPTER 6

I WANT TO DIE

FULL-LENGTH ICE BLANKETS DRAPE MY ENTIRE BODY, AND I'M SHAKING uncontrollably. The television is on. The 2004 Athens Olympics have begun, but I can't watch because of the cold. I glance toward the door, hoping for a nurse to remove the frigid blankets. Instead, two police officers stand there, casually talking and sipping coffee from paper cups.

A nurse arrives. She looks new, unfamiliar. I hope she notices that I'm cold and in pain. But I can't speak or indicate anything to her. "Brian, how are you feeling today?" she asks while placing her hand on my forehead. "Can you blink for me, sweetheart? Your parents told me that you were able to blink the other day. They were so excited."

I try to blink but can't. Shivering from this arctic chill, I watch her walk in and out of my room for what feels like forever. She finally returns and removes the icy blankets. What was the deal with that? Next thing I know, needles prick me. I see blood all over my left arm. I can't even imagine what's going to happen next.

Two other nurses roll in a portable cart with an assortment of cleaning supplies—shampoo, soap, towels. They push the table next to my bed, grab orange sponges, dip them in water, and start bathing me right in the bed. With water so tantalizingly close to my lips, I'm in a state of near delirium. The nurses obviously can't read my mind and I know I will remain parched, but their touch is soothing and refreshing. When was the last time I took a shower? Or more precisely, when was the last time I was given a sponge bath? The nurses tilt the bed so my head is closer to the floor than my feet. I'm getting a shampoo!

One nurse pours water over my hair and lathers in shampoo. Small drops of water splash on my face, mouth, lips. I struggle to slide my tongue out of my mouth and catch one of these falling drops of liquid goodness. Unfortunately, I have no luck, but my mouth is open a fraction for the breathing tube, and then out of nowhere, a water drop scores a direct hit!

The shampoo that they are using smells like strawberries. It takes me back to when I was in kindergarten and went to a farm and picked strawberries with my class. My mom and grandma were chaperones; it was a beautiful day and the sun was shining. I inhale the shampoo's fruity aroma because I know in a short while it will be gone, replaced by the sharp odor of rubbing alcohol.

The nurse rinses my hair with warm water, then dries it with a towel. My bed is set back to horizontal. My hair is combed, my fingernails and toenails trimmed. The two nurses lift me onto another table, replace my linens with a fresh set, and then move me back to the bed. The soft cool texture of the new sheets is pleasing.

While I'm pampered and fussed over, I listen to their conversation about the patient next door. It explains the two cops' presence. He's a convict who got jumped in prison when he left his cell. The attacker slammed his head into a brick wall. He now has severe brain damage.

The two nurses also discuss another gravely injured patient: a pregnant woman in her twenties who was stabbed by her husband. The knife tip broke off in her heart and she is listed in critical condition. The doctors are doing everything they can to save her, but her parents have been taking out their anger and frustration on the hospital staff and that is causing unnecessary interruptions. I can't imagine my parents ever acting this way around my doctors and nurses.

IT MIGHT BE THE NEXT DAY, BUT I CAN'T BE CERTAIN. MY DRY ACHING eyes have remained open for the entire time. I must have slept this way. Everything is blurred. I feel nauseous and feverish. I'm lying on my back, with a slight incline to the bed. I hear my dad's voice. Is he in my room? I don't see him.

A nurse sticks a needle in my arm, but I can't feel it as I usually do. She applies liquid solution to my eyes and my vision remains foggy and distorted. I still don't see my dad.

I begin to see a figure by the door wearing a blue T-shirt. It's Dad! I feel relieved. He's talking with a nurse. I overhear fragments of what they're discussing. Then two words—"bad news"—ambush me. They say a nasty infection has spread throughout my body. I now see my mom who looks more frightened than usual. The room begins to fill with big white fluffy clouds. I'm falling through them in a bright blue sky. I feel weightless in the bright sunshine, the breeze blowing through my hair. The white clouds are now turning gray and the sky has gotten darker, meaner. The room goes jet-black. My mind shuts down.

THE BED IS MOVING. I'M BEING ROLLED THROUGH THE HALLWAYS WITH several trailing pieces of medical equipment and IVs. We turn a corner and stop right before a set of folding doors. My eyes are rigid within their sockets. I'm drooling. This is no way to live. I sense bugs crawling all over my skin, biting me, trying to gnaw the flesh. My whole body feels like it's rotting away from the inside.

From my vantage point, I watch a revolving cast of nurses, doctors, hospital staff, and visitors walk by. Anyone who passes my bed rarely makes eye contact with me. Can you fault them? I must remind them of death. Best to ignore the corpse and keep on walking.

Then I'm wheeled into a cold room, with a big gray electronic machine. I remember this room. It's the CAT scan place. Because the bed is tilted, I finally get to see the machine. It looks intimidating, almost evil.

The nurses carefully flop me onto a table. The machine swallows me up again and the same robotic voice tells me to hold my breath for thirty seconds. I try to obey, but still no improvement. Several sluggish minutes go by and the scan is complete. I feel woozy as the machine returns me to the world. I vomit violently all over my gown, the table, and the floor. The female technician rushes to clean me. Is she the same woman who was here last time? Her perfume smells familiar, but before I can see her face, I'm wheeled into another room for X-rays.

Two nurses are talking right outside the room. I can hear them clearly. My name is brought up. One says that a doctor told her I'd probably be moved to a Baltimore nursing home for long-term care. The other nurse mentions that she had heard that too. Wait! Nursing home? And then it hits me as if somebody has just punched me in the face. Do doctors think that I will require twenty-four-hour care the rest of my life? Oh no, that can't be. Give or take a few broken bones and full paralysis, I'm doing all right. I can think, hear, smell, see. But what would I be like if I didn't have all those machines keeping me alive?

The brutal reality of my situation can't be glossed over. The machines in my hospital room are not for decorative purposes. Each one is playing a special role in allowing me to exist. Electricity *and* blood flow through my veins. Ten years ago, I wouldn't have even made it this far. But where exactly have I arrived? Those small, earlier signs of improvement, when I was able to blink and move my feet, now seem like false messages of hope. Being sentenced to permanent exile in a nursing home is worse than dying. I'd rather expire and have it end right here, right now.

I just turned eighteen. I was a good son, athlete, student, and friend to many. I never did drugs or drank alcohol on the weekends like most teenagers; I performed community service at my local church and Special Olympics. Whether I'm dead or living out the rest of my life in a nursing home, the outcome will be the same. I'll never know what it feels like to fall in love, get married, have a family. I'll never attend college. I'll never again get to swim in the ocean, take a walk with my dad, or have a long conversation with my mom. I'll never go outside, breathe the fresh air, see the blue sky and colorful sunsets.

I've held on for as long as I can. I've fought the good fight, yet it's just not enough. It's time to give up. As an athlete, you are taught *never* to quit. At swim practice, it was drilled into us. You train your body as you prepare your mind never to back off or surrender, especially in the heat of competition.

We aren't able to choose our destiny, but we can choose our reaction. Life can be beautiful, and it can also turn tragic in the tick of the clock or with a drop of rain on the windowsill. We are only here for a short time in this world. And my time is up. I'm ready to depart. I know what has to be done: I must shut down my will to live, and hope that my body obeys this final command. By doing so, I will finally find the peace that has eluded me. And when I go, I know that I will always be with my parents.

My nurses wheel me back to Room 19. As we move through the white hallways, my life starts to flash by. I'm assaulted by random fragmented memories ranging from when I was a little boy to the present, with each vision carrying a heavier emotional impact than the previous one.

As we approach my room, I see my parents standing by the door, talking with someone, a very large guy, the doctor. My parents look concerned. In reaction to whatever was said, my mom's mouth opens as if she is gasping for air. My dad places his arms around her. The doctor looks like he is trying to console both of them, and then walks away. Watching them from a short distance, I realize that I made a huge mistake wanting to die. I feel guilty for wanting to give up. My mom is sobbing behind a wad of tissues, but she won't look at me as I roll pass. My dad walks behind my bed, helping the nurses wheel in the rest of my equipment, IVs, and ventilator.

The nurses move the machines and medical equipment closer to me, reattaching tubes. The electronic symphony of beeping and buzzing resumes. Before the nurses leave the room, one of them injects some liquid into my left arm and attaches a new IV.

My dad approaches the left side of my bed, trying to force a smile that fails to mask his anxiety. It's almost like he peers into my soul and reads my thoughts. Has he stumbled upon my desire to die? He has a look of frantic desperation, like he has to do or say something before it's too late. But how did he know what I was thinking only minutes earlier?

He slides the aqua chair close to my bed, placing his hands over the wires and tubes that are connected to my chest, and crosses his arms. His head is bowed. "Brian, please stay strong. Keep fighting." He slowly gets up from his chair, pauses for several seconds, and walks over to my mom. "I don't want to do this," I hear my dad quietly say to her. "It's been a little over a month and a half and there's no real improvement. Not much progress at all. He's only getting worse. He's so tired; I don't think he has the strength to go on." I hear my mom sobbing.

Watching my parents suffer like this is much worse than being paralyzed and constantly being stabbed by needles and being left alone to rot in this bed, plagued by constant loneliness and everlasting confusion. I don't want to see my parents in perpetual anguish anymore. I can't leave them, but I can't continue like this either. Right now, I should be at a swim meet, being cheered on by them. As fate would have it, I'm being urged to keep going through the motions of living while stuck in my deathbed.

My dad walks back to me and sits down in the chair. My mom stays by the door where I can't see her. He stares blankly at the medical equipment. He struggles to speak. "Son, you have to be strong for us. We're almost out of the woods now; just a few more days, that is all it will take." He stands. There is frustration and anger in his voice as he paces around the room. "We want you to get out of this goddamn place!"

"Garth, please, calm down; you're scaring him," my mom interrupts in a startled voice.

"No, no, I can't, JoAnne. Chrissakes, I can't let this happen. He has to know that he has to keep fighting." He stands over my bed. "Son, I know you can hear me. Look at me! Now is the time. You are very sick. But dammit, I am not going to lose you! You can beat this; we know you can.

If I could switch places with you right now, I would do it in a heartbeat and you know that. We will get through it all together, but you have to make the choice to keep pushing through the pain. I know how tired you are, but please don't give up."

He walks to the bulletin board, his hands balled up in tense, clenched fists, looking at the photos. "Everyone is praying for you; everyone wants you to get out of this damn room and come home. They all want to see you."

He walks back over to my bed and sits down in the chair, slumped and defeated. His eyes are glazed and vacant. Is he thinking about what it's going to be like when I'm no longer in his life?

"You can do it, son." His voice is too choked to continue. As words fail him, a nurse enters the room and says that the visiting hour has ended.

My dad kisses me on my forehead. His parting words are, "We love you, and we will be back in a couple of hours." He asks my mom to say goodbye. She walks over to my bed. He's holding her up. She's unable to say anything, so she just holds my mitten-covered left hand, trembling and softly weeping.

CHAPTER 7

GARTH AND JOANNE BOYLE

MY PARENTS DON'T LOOK THE SAME TO ME. THEIR GESTURES ARE TWITCHY, nervous, awkward. Their blue eyes are bloodshot and puffy from sleepless nights. Dad's brown hair is going gray from stress. Mom's makeup is usually smudged from wiping away tears. They seem unsure how to approach me, what to say, how to act. They must be asking themselves, "Is that really our son lying there?"

As their only child, I was blessed by their generous attention. When I went to preschool, my parents would take turns during the week dropping me off in the mornings. I remember sitting at the window of that small school, madly bawling as I watched them get in their cars to leave for work. Every day we would go through this same routine, even though I knew that they would return in several hours.

I feel like that toddler now, waiting for them to rescue me, to take me home. They don't realize it, but they are bringing me back to life in a way that the most powerful medicine could never do. But will their devotion be strong enough to keep me alive? I can only hope that it does. It sounds selfish, but I can't imagine how life would be for them without me. We've always been best friends.

I have my mom's facial features and blonde hair and my dad's traits of hard work and self-discipline, but I also inherited their positive, outgoing outlook.

My dad was born in 1958 in Greensburg, Pennsylvania, a small town near Pittsburgh in the western part of the state. He was the youngest and scrappiest of seven children. His father was a concrete subcontractor in the construction industry. In 1962, my grandfather moved his family to Accokeek, Maryland, for better business opportunities in pouring concrete. Accokeek is a small town on the Potomac River located on the outskirts of Washington, D.C. At the time, it primarily consisted of sprawling horse farms and working-class people. My dad lived there for three years before his family moved to Oxon Hill, closer to the nation's capital.

My mom, born a year after my dad in Kansas City, Missouri, was the oldest of five children. Her father was a lieutenant in the Air Force and her family moved around a lot. When he made colonel, he was transferred to the Pentagon and moved to Oxon Hill with his family.

In the summer of 1970, my dad watched a moving van pull into the driveway across the street from his home, and that is when he saw my mom for the first time. She was moving into her family's new house. He thought she was the cutest girl he had ever seen. They were both eleven years old.

The town was small and their neighborhood was full of kids, so everyone hung out together, doing typical childhood stuff like softball, dodgeball, swimming, riding bikes, bowling, watching movies.

At thirteen, they were going steady, which continued through junior high and high school. During summers, she worked part-time after school at a day care center. My dad worked in the family construction business with his father and brothers. Weekends for the Boyle clan were spent at the beach at Ocean City, Maryland.

After graduation, Mom headed to college at Salisbury University, which was two hours away. Dad stayed with the family business, so he would drive down every weekend for visits. After four years, Mom graduated with a degree in business administration and began working for the U.S. Government at Bolling Air Force Base in Southwest Washington, D.C.

Two years later, they married. Not long afterward, I was born, on April 27, 1986, at 3:10 a.m. I weighed ten pounds, ten ounces, and I was twenty-two inches long. Dad always teased me about how my feet were hanging out of the newborn's bed because I was such a big baby. The same day I was born, NBC News was doing a special segment called "Healthy Babies" and they brought the cameras up to the maternity ward and filmed me being held by my mom.

I imagine that I was destined to like the water because at six weeks, my parents dipped my tiny toes into the Atlantic. When I was ten, our family spent two weeks in Oahu. Our hotel was near the famous Waikiki beach. From our balcony, I could see Diamondhead. There were many surfers riding the waves. I said to my parents, "Let's go swimming!" I rented a bodyboard and my dad went with a surfboard, which I thought was cool. I watched him paddle out about two hundred yards in the water to join the surfers. It was only his second time on a surfboard, but he was determined to sample the Hawaiian surf.

My dad and I were always involved in sports—hitting baseballs at the local batting cage, playing tennis, one-on-one basketball, going to the golf driving range, running, riding bikes, swimming, playing catch with the football. Whatever kind of activity we did, there was always a hint of competition. He was really fit from all the heavy lifting that he did at work. I always wanted to have his big arms and shoulders.

My parents didn't idly sit at home. We took day trips to the capital and Baltimore for visits to the museums, zoos, and art galleries. Music was always a big deal in our house too, and my dad's record collection was impressive. I would spend hours sitting in front of the turntable and cassette player listening to Led Zeppelin, AC/DC, Foghat, Van Halen, Mötley Crüe, INXS, Rod Stewart, Jimi Hendrix, Neil Young, The Cure, Fleetwood Mac, Bob Marley and the Wailers, The Beastie Boys, The Gap Band, and Prince.

When I was in second grade, we moved to the small town of Welcome in the rural part of southern Maryland because my parents liked its tranquility. Welcome's claim to fame is that it's part of Charles County. In April of 1865, John Wilkes Booth escaped through the county after shooting president Abraham Lincoln. He was on his way to Virginia. With its Civil War heritage and picturesque beauty, Welcome is an ideal place to raise a family. It's only two minutes from the Potomac River. Our home sits on a big hill in the woods.

Meanwhile, my father's family concrete business was doing well. He worked on projects at the U.S. Capitol, Redskins Stadium, the MCI Center, Whitehurst Freeway, Union Station, and the FDR Memorial. Because of his job, my mom and I rarely got to see him except on weekends. So he made a big decision: he left the family business and joined forces with another concrete firm close to home. New housing developments were booming in southern Maryland.

My mom also transferred from the Air Force to work for the Navy at the Patuxent River Naval Base in the next county.

Then, the first big tragedy struck our family. It was 1992. We were spending the weekend in Ocean City. Dad looked thin, unhealthy. When he was wearing a bathing suit, his ribs were prominently showing; he had lost a lot of weight. He was always muscular, so this seemed odd. He was thirty-three years old. A week later, he went to the family doctor, thinking he had ruptured a hernia on a job site. His physician ran some tests, then recommended he see a urologist. Two days later, the urologist told him that there was a strong possibility he had a cancerous tumor in his right testicle and that he would need immediate surgery to remove it. Back then, whenever the word *cancer* was used, it meant an automatic death sentence. Only the year before, his father had died from prostate cancer. Now I was going to lose my dad, too.

I avoided my dad when he came home from the hospital, because I thought he was going to leave me forever. I was just six years old. On the fourth day, he got out of bed for the first time. He could barely stand up, let alone walk, but he somehow made it to the bottom of the stairs, hunched over and holding onto the banister for support with both hands. He was in agony, looking like a crippled ninety-year-old man. He saw me at the top of the stairs looking down. He could see that I was frightened. As our eyes met, he let go of the railing, stood straight up, and smiled, letting me know that I could count on him.

Now it's my turn, in this bed, in Room 19, to show that same kind of strength. I have to let my parents know that I'm not going anywhere, either.

CHAPTER 8

THE SMILE

When my parents come back for the afternoon visiting hour, I need to let them know how much I love them. With enough concentration and effort, I can blink, but that's not enough. I have to try something else. Then it dawns on me: I can smile. That would be perfect! But how am I going to get my facial muscles to cooperate?

I try to find awareness in my lips but they are numb. I keep searching for sensation, a slight twitch or quiver. Fifteen minutes go by, and I'm sweating terribly, my body seems on fire. Finally, I'm able to purse my lips. I'm growing weak from the strain, but I can't give up.

I press my lips together to get the nerves in my lips and mouth active again. I feel blood rushing through the area. I repeat the puckering, but I'm starting to feel nauseous. Yet I won't stop until I have created a smile.

I focus attention on the tiny muscles behind my lips, but there's no motion from the start. This is going to be an even bigger challenge. I always took the ability to smile for granted. I go back to the kissing motion, trying to loosen the muscles.

I have to take a break. I stare at the ceiling, trying to gather inspiration, anything that will help me succeed. I think about the reaction my parents will have when they see me smiling. I return to the kissing motion, and out of nowhere I feel like I'm zapped with a thousand volts of electricity. My body goes into a violent seizure. The machines in my room begin to blare. Several nurses hurry to my side.

After several minutes, my body is finally released from this horror spell. The room is spinning. Foam spews from my mouth. I can barely see. The machines' alarms have quieted and returned to their normal beeping and pinging. I hear the nurses ask one another what could have caused my seizure. One suggests that they need to check with a neurologist to see if I have brain damage. As she runs out of the room to find him, the other four nurses stay with me. One nervously gives me an injection. She holds the needle very cautiously, hoping that I don't start shaking again because that could pose a risk of breaking the needle off in a vein.

I lie there on my side, breathing hard. The nurses are gently rubbing my forehead and softly dabbing off the sweat with a small damp towel. My dad's voice from earlier replays constantly in my head: "I know how tired you are, but please don't give up."

I stubbornly seek out sensations in my lips once more, trying to strengthen them to create a simple smile. Even if I have another seizure, I will keep trying. I push my lips together and release them. I do this several times before I'm zapped again, my body flailing about. There's a sudden sharp pain in my groin, and the arm restraints loosen from all the wild motion. The nurses struggle to keep me flat on the bed. My body continues to convulse and the room starts to turn dark, when I see the nurse come back with the neurologist and an ICU doctor. They join the nurses in helping to calm me down, while they analyze the situation. When I go limp, the nurses rush to strap my arms down to the bed, this time binding them more tightly.

One of the nurses notices that the sheets by my legs are wet. She pulls off the cover to see what happened. "Oh dear," I hear her say, "Brian just wet the bed. There's urine everywhere. His thrashing must have dislodged the catheter when he was having his seizure. Aw, poor guy, that must have really hurt!"

As the nurses roll me about on the bed, switching the sheets and giving me a new gown, I listen to the neurologist tell the ICU doctor that he's worried about possible brain damage. He thinks I need an MRI, X-rays, and brain scans so they can figure out what's wrong.

The nurses quickly gather all my machines and IVs and rapidly wheel me out of the room. They push me down the hallways at a much faster pace than usual. I watch the ceiling lights flicker past. I'm wheeled into the radiology department, where I first encountered the perfumed woman.

While waiting to be shoved into the big white machine, I try to move my lips. They are sore. I concentrate on lip puckering. It's so difficult. I flex my cheeks a little bit, but there is no movement. I also try to move my eyes around, just to get everything working together. The eyelids flutter at first, and then surprisingly they break free from their frozen-straight-ahead position.

I keep moving my lips back and forth, flexing, squeezing, relaxing, until I sense another seizure about to commence. My body is thrown into a bucking spasm and the nurses rush over to my bed. A flurry of hands struggles to calm my body down. This seizure only lasts about thirty seconds. I watch the nurses wipe sweat from their faces.

I'M BACK IN ROOM 19. A NURSE INJECTS ME WITH SOME KIND OF medication in a new IV that she has just inserted into my left forearm.

A second nurse takes blood from my other forearm. I feel like a human dartboard.

I move my tongue around the inside of my mouth. For the first time, I feel some sensation in my jaw and cheeks. Determined, I try twitching, but nothing. Only after the tenth time am I finally able to generate a response, and that's all it takes to fuel the next attempt, and then the next. I keep at it. One, two, three, four, five . . . and then I have to rest. The muscles in my face are rapidly tiring from all the activity. My face feels like it has a cramp.

I rest for a little while, and then my body tenses up. *Please not again, not now!* My body explodes in a wild fit of tossing, but this time I try to stay rigid. My teeth grind and foam churns in my mouth. *Stay focused*, I keep thinking. *Just let it pass and run its course.* The seizure soon subsides and I'm finally released from its powerful hold. I'm drenched in a cold sweat.

This episode drains my last remaining energy. All I can do now is take a long breather, conserving strength for my parents' arrival.

I close my eyes and begin to daydream. I'm a little boy again, out in the front yard in the driveway on a warm spring day. My dad just got home from work, and I run out to see him and give him a hug. I'm happy to see him. After he goes in the house to say hello to my mom, he comes back outside and we throw the football. "Go long, Brian. Go all the way out past the tree in the middle of the driveway," he yells as I toss the ball to him and start to run down the driveway. I get to the end of the driveway, and as soon as I turn around, the ball lands right between my hands.

"Good throw, Dad, but watch this!" I throw it back to him and watch him standing there, as he is getting ready to catch it. We throw it back and forth, as the sun starts going down behind the trees, casting shadows along the driveway.

I open my eyes, reflecting on the memory. But something about my face feels different. There's tightness around my cheeks and mouth. Could I be doing what I think I'm doing? I remember that feeling! I haven't felt this in ages. I'm finally smiling! I can't believe it! Tears fill my eyes with a sense of accomplishment.

I hear footsteps outside my room. My mom and dad enter, both of them wearing a sad look of despair. My dad sees me first. The stress in his face immediately disappears when he notices me smiling. "JoAnne, look! Look!" he shouts. "He's smiling—can you believe it?"

Several nurses rush in, wondering what's wrong. I watch their jaws drop.

Mom and Dad walk toward me, not saying anything. They're gleaming with happiness. Both stare in amazement. I continue looking up at them, smiling.

The smile is everything I hoped it would be. It is so much more than a common facial gesture that I had once taken for granted; it is a defining gesture, a pure expression of love that has brought my parents and me out of the depths of the deepest darkness.

CHAPTER 9

THE KISS

I'M JUST WAKING UP WHEN I HEAR A WOMAN'S VOICE THAT APPARENTLY exists outside of any dream. "Brian, can you hear me?" I'd like to continue sleeping, but I feel someone tapping my chest as if knocking on a door. I open my eyes to find out what is happening.

Temporarily blinded by the room's brightness, I see a small woman in a white lab coat standing on the left-hand side of my bed.

"There you are, Brian, good morning. My name is Dr. Kulkarni, and I work in physical medicine and rehabilitation. I heard from your nurses that you were able to smile yesterday. They even said that you could blink. Is this true?"

Without thinking, I shut my eyes, because I want to go back to sleep. But I then hurry to reopen my eyes. Why can't I just keep them shut? At least the chest tapping has stopped.

"That's wonderful—that blink. I'm here because I want you to perform some very minimal tasks. We're going to start your physical therapy, and this is an evaluation to see what you're capable of."

One of my nurses comes in the room and walks near my bed as Dr. Kulkarni continues talking. The nurse takes a tubelike device and starts fiddling around with my breathing tube, which causes me to cough up the fluid blockage collected in my fragile lungs.

Dr. Kulkarni watches patiently as the nurse finishes cleaning out the gooey lung buildup. The nurse then inserts a new IV into my arm, and gives me "breakfast" through the drip feed tube that travels down my nose into my stomach.

"Can you smile for me?" Dr. Kulkarni asks in a curious tone. I try but am too weak to manage anything substantial. But she at least notices a hint of something. "Good job," she says after the muscles in my face go slack again.

She walks over to my right side, holding a clipboard in her hand. She places her left hand under my right hand and raises it about an inch off the bed.

"Can you squeeze my hand?" she asks. I struggle to move my fingertips and wrap them around her hand. "Very good," she says as she walks over to the left-hand side of my bed. She picks up my left hand and gives the same request. There's no sensation in my left hand; it's completely numb. "That's okay, don't worry. We were thinking this would happen, since your left shoulder suffered a lot of nerve damage from your accident, but you'll be able to move it in a few years, and there's a really good chance that you'll have full recovery, too."

A few years? What? She can't be right, can she?

She's busy writing stuff down on her clipboard, and then walks to the end of my bed. "Can you wiggle your toes?"

I try to focus my attention where my toes are attached, and once the mind-body connection is made, my toes move slightly.

"Now how about your feet? I'm going to put pressure on the front of your feet and I want you to push them forward. Okay?"

I stop wiggling my toes and try to push my feet forward. My ankles make a slight crackling noise and then a pop, and they move forward about half an inch. I try again and my feet move forward about an inch. "That's great," she says.

She then walks over to the left side of the room. I'm not sure what she is doing, though I hear her fiddling with some type of medical instruments. I try to move my head so I can see better, but my head can only rotate about an inch to the left, which is still an accomplishment, because yesterday I couldn't move my head at all.

She walks back to my bed, pushing a little trolley with a machine that has a system of wires. A handheld remote-control gizmo lies next to it. "This is the last thing I'm going to do today," she explains in a sympathetic voice. "This test is called an electromyogram and it will let me and your physical therapists know how your nerves and muscles are functioning and responding." She pauses, and then picks up the remote-control device from the cart. "So what I'm going to do is send an electrical impulse to certain areas of your body to see if we can get a response. You may feel a slight amount of pressure that will be uncomfortable, but it will be over soon." I like everything she just said, except the part about it being uncomfortable.

She applies a jellylike substance to various areas of my arms, legs, and shoulders. She brings the handheld device closer to my right arm. She presses a button and my arm jerks from the electrical shock. *Whoa, please don't do that again*, I silently beg. She zaps my right leg and it automatically lifts off the bed several inches. This feels like torture. After several minutes of being zapped, I stare blankly at the ceiling.

"See, now that wasn't so bad, was it?" she says to me in a cheerful voice. Is she serious?

She walks over to one of my nurses, whom I don't recognize, standing just outside my room and filling out a stack of paperwork. I can just barely hear their conversation because of the distance. Dr. Kulkarni asks her if I am able to speak. The nurse briefly looks my way. "Well, we really don't know yet," I hear her say. "There was evidence of a massive concussion from the crash. The fact that he's still living is a miracle. He has been through so much already for the past month and a half. He had an incident a few weeks ago where his tracheotomy tube clogged up and he couldn't breathe for several minutes. The lack of oxygen for his brain may have had a catastrophic effect. If he is able to speak one day, then that will be fantastic, but his overall mental capacity, if and when he comes out of the coma, is unknown."

Huh? This latest overheard news alert sends me furiously spiraling into panic mode. My heart is racing while trying to keep pace with my out-of-control thoughts. I have been here for a month and a half? How is that possible? I only remember waking up just a few days ago. Why did my parents tell me that I only had a few broken bones and that I would be out of here in a few days? Are they just trying to sugarcoat the fact that I might have suffered brain damage? This just doesn't seem possible, because I'm thinking right now; I seem coherent. Don't these people know I'm blinking on command and trying to smile and wiggle my toes? Isn't that good enough evidence that my brain is working like it's always worked, except that I can't speak? And if I can't get words to come out of my mouth, I will just have to learn sign language once I get more feeling back in my fingers. Whatever got me in this mess—and I still don't know what accident everyone is referring to—I will not have it defeat me. Still, six weeks of my life have been excised like a giant tumor. Is this what amnesia is like? Or maybe I do have brain damage. I'm more scared than I have ever been in my life.

After she gathers up her instruments and clipboard, Dr. Kulkarni leaves the room. A nurse walks in right afterward. I move my eyes in her direction to see if I recognize her and I do. She's smiling and is happy to see me. "Hi Brian, I'm Nurse Kimberly. Do you remember me?" I blink once in response. She looks over the gauges on my monitors and machines. She attaches a new bag of fluid for my IV, removes blood for testing, cleans out the buildup in my breathing tube, checks my catheter, wraps air-filled compression braces around my legs, and turns on the television. I tilt my head so I can see the screen. There's a news program about the Iraq War on, and the screen is full of wounded soldiers and civilian victims from a mass suicide bombing.

I hear the water running in the sink and immediately start obsessing about getting a drink, just one lousy sip. It's incredible how parched my throat feels.

I glance up at the clock. It is 10:43. I watch the second hand go around and around, every sixty seconds marking a different drink in my imagination. For the first minute, it's a tall glass of ice-cold water. The next minute, it's one of those plastic two-liter bottles of Mountain Dew that I used to consume in one long continuous gulp. And wouldn't it be great if I could swim in a pool of lemon-lime Gatorade and take a drink every time I put my head below the surface? Then it's onto ice-cold milk—so cold that it's right at the threshold of freezing. Of course, I can't leave out fruit juices—apple, orange, cranberry, pineapple. I'm so desperate for liquid salvation that even a sip from a puddle of dirty water would be a treat. Thinking about all the refreshing possibilities causes me to drool. Kimberly wipes my mouth off with a small towel.

Kimberly walks over and turns the volume of the television up. She begins to giggle. I look up at the television to see what she thinks is so funny. It's a talk show and there is a blonde woman walking out on stage and waving to the audience. I squint to see if I have seen this show before and then realize that it's Ellen DeGeneres. I've always been a big fan of Ellen's talk show and her sitcoms. She starts dancing on stage. Her positive energy pumps up the audience. Watching Ellen, I've stopped thinking about being so thirsty.

Engrossed with Ellen, I almost don't see my parents enter the room. They seem more relieved and less sad. My dad is carrying a small blue paper bag, and my mom is actually walking without a nurse holding her arm. She is clenching a tissue, but she is not crying. My dad asks me to blink and smile. I do both right away. He puts his fingers under my right hand and tells me to squeeze and I do. He then tells me to shake his hand, and I softly move his hand a few inches up and down.

He pulls the chair with the aqua cushion close to my bed and sits down. My mom stands on the right side of the bed. My dad says that he brought some of my favorite CDs, including the Omaha, Nebraska, rock band 311, along with a small foam globe. He says that by squeezing it several times a day, it will help reactivate the nerves and muscles in my hands that have been placed on standby. He gives the ball to my mom who places it in my right hand. I squeeze it a few times, which pleases them.

Kimberly walks in the room and greets my parents, then rechecks the various machines and monitors. When she's done, she leaves. The Boyle family watches *Ellen* together. A little bit later, Kimberly comes back into my room. Following right behind her is another nurse who is pushing a stretcherlike table. It's Victoria who gave me the sponge bath. My dad helps the two nurses position the contraption next to my bed.

The next thing I know, I am lifted onto this table. A soft dark red cushion covers it. Kimberly explains, "Brian, the table you're laying on now is actually a chair and what we are going to do is tilt you up so your body gets used to sitting upright again. You've been on your back for quite a long time, so now we are going to gradually transition you to being upright because it is going to take some getting used to."

Both nurses strap a safety restraint belt around my waist, tie my arms and legs down to both sides of the table, and gradually bring me forward. Pressure immediately builds in my lower back. My butt feels like it's sitting on razors. The pain is intense. How long am I going to have to sit like this? I rapidly blink to get their attention, but they don't understand what I'm trying to say.

All of a sudden, my body spasms from the excruciating pain. The seizure arrives with a frightening fury, throwing my limbs out of control. My mom screams in shock and darts out of the room while my dad looks on in horror. My mouth is spewing red foam and saliva. Right before I vomit, the room goes all black as if someone has flicked a switch and mercifully cast me into darkness.

I'm still stuck in an inclined position in this chair. The nausea hasn't gone away. The room is spinning and I instantly throw up; disgusting vomit covers my hospital gown and bare arms and legs. The aggressive reflex from throwing up forces out the feeding tube that goes from my nose to my stomach. A nurse rushes into my room and cleans up the mess, changes my gown, and then leaves. Less than a minute later, she returns with a doctor who says that I now need another operation to replace the feeding tube. Why did I have to wake up and vomit?

MORNING. THE OLD FEEDING TUBE IS CURLED INSIDE A PLASTIC BAG waiting to be picked up. Long, black, and thin, it reminds me of a snake being threaded deep inside my gut.

My parents visit at eleven o'clock and we watch *Ellen*. When their visiting session ends, I nod and smile. I even wave goodbye with my right arm that I'm now able to raise about a foot and a half off of the bed. Right after they depart, I'm wheeled to the operating room to insert a new feeding tube. My typical entourage of ventilator, IVs, and various machines accompanies me through the hospital corridors.

A kindhearted nurse named Debbie tells me that the operation is going to be extremely uncomfortable. Her words elevate my stress. She says that the doctor will be inserting the tube into my nose and threading it all the way through my throat until it reaches my stomach. Special care must be taken to ensure that it does not pass through the windpipe and down into my lungs. The tube's insertion must be done without anesthesia, so I need to be awake the entire time. Seeking to bolster my spirits, Debbie says that it would be great if I could blow my mom a kiss when I return from surgery.

I'm wheeled into a cold room where I'm positioned directly underneath a large X-ray machine. The doctor arrives and says he's ready to begin. I'm not. I dread this procedure, so I shut my eyes as if I have the power to block out the imminent unpleasantness. Debbie holds my hand.

I feel the tube entering my nose, creating a faint tickling sensation followed by intense pressure in my nasal cavity. The tube winds down my throat, causing a fierce gagging reflex. "I have to back up and retrace my steps, because the tube is going down the wrong path," says the doctor regretfully. He pulls it out about four inches and then starts down a different path. He stops again, pauses for a few seconds, pulls the tube back out about two inches, and pushes it back in forcefully creating a loud popping noise. This is pure agony. I stare at my tormenter, begging for his mercy. He answers my nonvocal pleading and tapes the end of the tube to my nose.

I continue to lie there on the operating table, drenched in a clammy sweat. Debbie strokes my forehead. She offers congratulations for being brave, but courage is the last emotion I feel right now. I'm totally spent, my vision reduced to a foggy haze.

When I return to my room, the reward for enduring that awful encounter with the feeding tube is another upright session in what I now call the "angry chair." I hate this chair. I almost wish that I were back in the operating room.

After what feels like ten minutes, my lower body starts turning numb. After thirty minutes, I'm drooling. After an hour, I'm sweating rapidly and feel an intense discomfort in my lungs. I hear the ventilator working harder than usual to pump air into my weak lungs.

I watch ICU visitors walk by my room. If they happen to look inside, they will see a motionless, drooling person strapped to a chair. *Poor damaged soul,* they must think, walking away in revulsion.

Debbie enters my line of sight from the left side of the room; she must have been sitting behind me the whole time. I look at her with my eyes wide open, trying to show her that I want out of the angry chair. She says, "Okay, twenty minutes is up. Let's take a break, and we'll try sitting for thirty minutes in a few hours. Sound good?"

I want to scream. Twenty minutes! That's all that was? This is absurd, but at least I get to lie back down in bed.

Debbie and one of the hospital staff remove the restraints from the chair and they carefully transfer me back to my bed. I wiggle the fingers on my right hand and feel the cool texture of the white sheets. My bed is positioned at a slight incline. Debbie places the blue foam ball in my right hand and I start squeezing it. I have grown used to this small ball, which reminds me of Wilson, Tom Hanks's volleyball and sole companion in *Cast Away*.

My parents walk into the room, grinning. I wait until my mom is looking right at me. I then slowly launch my right arm straight up, touching my lips, before it loses its battle with gravity and drops back down. She looks totally surprised. Debbie claps her hands in joy. "You did it! You blew your mom a kiss!"

CHAPTER 10

THROWING THE DISCUS

I WONDER IF SOMEONE CAN ACTUALLY PERISH FROM BOREDOM. HOW DO prisoners locked away in solitary confinement manage to maintain their mental clarity without going crazy? When it's just you and your runaway thoughts keeping you company, it's not like you can find pleasant distractions like reading or conversation to ward off the emptiness. I desperately want to break out of this jail that is my body. Can I ever become the old Brian? Will I ever stretch my legs in our backyard, swim in a cold lake, attend a rock concert?

Each morning, nurses strap me into the angry chair, positioning my body so it can sit upright at a thirty-degree angle. This is supposed to improve blood flow in my legs. While I feel less like a corpse when I'm confined in the angry chair than lying in bed, I only wish I could tell the nurses to loosen the restraining belts which are cutting off the circulation in my chest, waist, and legs. The way they have me strapped down, I feel like a catatonic patient in a mental institution.

Sitting like this, my paralyzed left arm dangles uselessly by my side, while my right arm rests inert upon my chest like I should be reciting the Pledge of Allegiance. The fingers on my right hand look foreign and small, just paper-thin skin stretched tightly around the bones. They remind me of illustrations of skeletal fingers in my high school biology textbook. I wonder if my entire body is skin and bones. I must have lost a lot of weight. Exactly how much?

Not long ago, I weighed 230 pounds. My weight changed according to the sports I played: swimming on the high school team in the winter and, in the spring, throwing the discus and putting the shot for the track team. I always had difficulty with this transition because swimming requires leanness and the field events require power and mass. In swimming, I tried to stay at 180 pounds, just right for my height of five feet and eleven inches. When track season started, I'd quickly gain 50 pounds by drinking a lot of protein shakes. I didn't want to be big, but I had to be this size if I wanted to compete with other discus throwers in Maryland. I was one of the smallest throwers because most of them were burly linebackers who played football in the fall. Some weighed 300 pounds.

If I couldn't match their size and strength, my weapon was extreme foot speed. Since I had a much smaller frame, I was able to spin around at a much higher velocity. That is one of the most important factors in achieving height and distance when heaving the discus.

I remember one track and field meet near the end of the season of my senior year. My teammate and good friend Sean Thompson had been virtually undefeated in shot put and discus since we started throwing together in our freshman year. He had college track scholarships to pretty much anywhere he wanted to go. Naturally, I had a burning desire to beat him one day. I had plans of swimming in college, but I still wanted to outthrow Sean just once.

Sean and I were doing our warm-ups when the throwing judge blew his whistle for us to begin. I continued to practice my technique and do some push-ups to get the blood pumping. Sean was up first. He let out a thundering yell as he hurled the metal disc out into the grassy infield. When it landed, a big clump of dirt and grass flung upward. It was a good, decent throw, but not one of his best.

I sat on a small hill away from everyone, waiting for my turn to throw. I felt the hot sun on my face and arms, and I smelled sunscreen in the slight breeze. I took a sip of Mountain Dew from its green plastic bottle. I held the discus in my right hand, feeling the cool metal on my palm and fingertips. I rubbed my hand in the dirt next to my feet and felt the discus's dull edges to make sure I could get a good grip on it when I threw it. I placed my hand on the center, spreading my fingers wide. I pulled my index finger back so there was a space between my fingers to maximize the grip. I tossed the three-pound, nine-ounce disc a few inches up in the air, causing it to rotate several times before landing back between the ends of my fingers.

The throwing judge called my name. I walked around the fenced-in barrier onto the concrete platform, and then into the circle. I took a deep breath for clarity, slowly exhaling as I shrugged my shoulders forward, getting in one last stretch. I did a quick practice spin and then aligned my feet at the top of the circle, visualizing the form and technique needed to throw as far as possible. I felt the disc's weight in my hand, gripping it with my fingers and palm. I stood on my toes as I rotated my body as far back as it could travel, gaining momentum, spinning around as fast as I could, and launched the discus into the bright blue sky. After my body came to a stop, I watched the thin metal object slice through the air like a tiny spaceship flying off into the sky. It landed just a few feet short of Sean's throw, and a surge of adrenaline flowed through me.

I walked out of the circle and around the fence, glancing over at Sean to see his reaction. A look of concern was hidden behind his artificial smile. Secretly, I knew he was cursing my existence under his breath.

After several minutes, the rest of the throwers took their turn in the circle, and then the second of three rounds began. I did a few quick drills over in the grass. It was Sean's turn, and he launched the orb about ten feet past his first throw. He lifted his arms up in the air in victory, and I gave him a high five as I made my way into the circle.

I went through the same motions, but this time the throw felt different. As I rotated, I'm not exactly sure what happened, but I was able to obtain more speed and the angle of release achieved the ideal plane. I watched the discus soar, landing a few inches further than Sean's spot and nearly four feet past my personal record of 145 feet.

I couldn't believe what I had just accomplished, the culmination of thousands of throws I had done in practice and meets over the past four years. I walked over to my coach, Mr. Covey, who shook my hand and gave me a hug. Sean couldn't top my throw in his final attempt, so I won the event. My athletic dream came true.

But that satisfying memory is eclipsed by Room 19's reality. I can't even toss a pencil in the air or snap my fingers. A wave of rage crashes inside my head. My body, in response, reacts by shaking ferociously, trying to wriggle itself free from the restraints. But I am too weak, so nothing happens. I slam my head against the chair's top in agitated fury and grind my teeth, shredding my tongue, to feel something other than numbness. Blood dribbles out of my mouth and down my chin.

"Calm down, Brian," says a nurse, rushing over. "It's going to be okay. You're getting better; things are improving. You just have to relax and be patient." Somehow I gather the strength to move my right hand away from my chest and allow it to hang limply by my side. I can't bear to look at my former discus throwing hand anymore.

DESPITE EVERYTHING, I NEED TO START THINKING LIKE AN OPTIMIST. Looking back at my physical therapy sessions, which began three days ago, I can see I've made visible progress. I can do the absolute basics—smile, blink, and squeeze hands. To someone of normal health, these activities would be considered infantile. But in a way, I'm relearning everything just like a baby. I keep thinking how this is affecting my parents. They are my inspiration. I can't let them down now. I'm close to returning to the world of the living again.

If I could only speak, I'd be able to leave behind this locked-in existence. I'd tell my parents that their son is a fighter. I'd thank the nurses and doctors for all the hard work it took to keep me going. I'd ask for a glass of water. I'd tell my physical therapist that I don't like being awakened at six in the morning by having my chest tapped with her hand. I'd tell strangers in the hospital corridor who stare at me in fright to look away! I'd ask the nurse for a blanket when I'm cold. I'd tell my parents to take me outside in a gurney or wheelchair.

Regaining the ability to talk is the key that will unlock my dungeon's door. Yet whenever I try saying anything, no sound comes out. Even when I attempt to mouth words, no one understands what I want to say. Nurses and doctors always react with the same puzzled look.

Talking seems easy to do. Just exhale some air from your lungs, move your tongue and lips a little here and there, and you create syllables and, from there, words, and then entire sentences. I can't even say "Daddy" or "Mama" like most one-year-olds. How long will I remain voiceless? The rest of my life? Why can't anyone hear me?

CHAPTER 11

"HELLO"

I'M IN THE ANGRY CHAIR WHEN THE NURSE NAMED DEBBIE COMES INTO my room. She says that she is going to try to get me to speak. I blink to let her know that I understand, and I blink again with a faint smile to let her know that I'm excited. She is going to insert a small clear catheter into the hub of the tracheostomy tube at the base of my throat. This procedure will force me to cough, which is when I'm supposed to say something. It seems simple enough. I hope the process works.

The tube tickles and scrapes my throat. Rather than cough, I gag. My eyes begin to tear up, while my breathing turns heavy with the pain. I don't want Debbie to try again; there has to be another way of getting me to speak. But she can't know what I'm thinking, and so, with kind, motherly assurance, she places her hand on my chest to calm me down. Several minutes later, she reinserts the tube, and this time I'm able to stifle the gag reflex and make a faint gurgling noise.

Debbie attempts several more times but she's becoming tired. She's also concerned about my discomfort. She pauses, wiping away beads of sweat that have collected on her forehead. "You can do it. Just say something, even a few letters will do." The only noise coming from my throat is raspy, gargling coughing. It sounds animal-like, not human. After several more tries, Debbie finally takes a much-needed break. It's hard to tell which one of us is more exhausted.

She delicately pulls the device out of the breathing tube opening and lets me rest. I blink rapidly to let her know we should continue. Debbie walks to the other side of the room and quietly says to another nurse named Faye, "Do you really think he is even capable of talking again?"

I sure can! I want to shout. *Please don't give up on me. Come on— give me one more chance. I'm getting the hang of it. I know I am.* But maybe Debbie is right. This realization drains me of hope. *You moron! You were given the chance to talk and you blew it!* My head droops forward in despair. I feel defeated and ashamed.

I then notice a group of people approaching my room. It's Dr. Catevenis leading a small group of people in white lab coats. They all look to be in their mid-to-late twenties. Medical students? Interns? They gather around my bed. Dr. Catevenis explains to them how proud he is of my progress. I want to hide under the bed. These strangers are staring at me like I'm a caged, wounded animal.

Dr. Catevenis asks if I can say hello to his group. I slowly lift my right arm and wave my hand, welcoming them to my cell. I even add a faint smile for hospitality's sake. It's always important to be a gracious host.

I study the reactions of these young doctors, but can't read their expressions. Or rather, I see nothing on their faces. Just stone. No returned greeting or acknowledgment, not even a small nod. Here I am, lingering half-alive between human and machine, but I still can express empathy and kindness. Yet all I receive from these young doctors are vacant stares. I'm nothing but an anonymous body to them, perhaps someone they might read about one day in medical journals. I feel sorry for their future patients. I want them all to leave.

Dr. Catevenis concludes his brief talk by saying, "You're doing good Brian; keep it up, buddy. I will be back to check on you soon." A good, thoughtful, and considerate physician, he gives me a thumbs-up gesture and leads away his young charges.

Debbie returns with another small clear plastic tube to help me speak. Fantastic! This is my big chance to redeem myself. When the tube is reinserted, I cough violently. My lungs rattle and crackle, but the sensation seems different, with the coughing more rhythmic. Way down in my lungs, a pocket of air develops, rising up through me like a geyser. I feel a word forming, and I see Dr. Catevenis walking around the corner. He stops right in front of my room, and the long-awaited moment takes place before his very eyes.

"Hello," I announce in a scratchy voice. I want to say more but the attempt fizzles in a drawn-out hissing.

"Brian, you did it!" he says in complete astonishment. "You're talking!"

That word, "hello," I know is just the start of more to come. One day I will put entire sentences together.

Debbie is doing a gleeful jig. She hugs Dr. Catevenis. Several nurses come into my room. Everyone is beaming. It feels like a party. I want to add to the merriment and proclaim, *Thank you everyone for keeping me alive*. But for now, that lone "hello" will have to suffice.

DEBBIE, WITH THE HELP OF ANOTHER NURSE, MOVES ME BACK TO THE bed. She reattaches a few IVs and checks to make sure my catheter is in place. She turns on the television and places the remote control next to my ear. The remote has speakers built into it. NBC is showing highlights from the 2004 Olympics in Athens. I look forward to watching the swimming.

As much as I love watching them, I admit to harboring jealousy toward these Olympic athletes. Here they perform on the world stage, healthy men and women, doing what they love, representing their countries and living their dreams. I was also an athlete. Now my sole competition is with my body. The Athens athletes are concerned about going faster, higher, stronger than their peers. Me? Don't I deserve a gold medal for saying my first word?

DEBBIE FINISHES HER DAY SHIFT AND SAYS GOODBYE. I LOOK AT HER and smile and slightly nod my head. She is such a nice woman. Before she goes, she asks me if I need anything. I direct my eyes toward the radio, and she knows right away what I want. She turns it on. I give her a thumbs-up in gratitude. The song playing is "Rooster," by Alice in Chains, one of my all-time favorite songs. As soon as I hear the music, my body is temporarily in a state of total peace, almost as if I'm back to my old self again. I silently sing along with the lyrics: *Ain't found a way to kill me yet* . . . This song neatly defines who I am, in this bed, in this hospital room.

TONY WALKS INTO MY ROOM. HE'S MY RESPIRATORY THERAPIST. I LIKE him. He has a dark complexion, is bald, and has a gentle but motivating personality. He says that everyone is talking about how I said my first word. He examines my tracheostomy tube. "Okay, so what I'm going to do is pick up where Debbie left off," he says. "I talked it over with the doctors, and we decided to try an alternative method of having you speak. I think you'll probably like it better." He's addressing me as if I'm a dog, not truly capable of fully understanding what he's saying.

After he removes the yucky fluid buildup in my lungs, he carefully places a small buttonlike piece of equipment on the outer hub of the tracheostomy tube. The one-way valve, he tells me, will open to let air in when I breathe. The valve closes during exhaling, causing air to leave and permitting speech.

He steps back several feet. I nervously open my mouth and exhale. In amazement, several words come sputtering out of my mouth in a distorted high-pitched sound. "Hello, Tony . . . oh my God, I am talking! I am actually talking! Can you believe it?" Tony looks dumbfounded. He runs out of the room, grabbing nurses and pushing them into my room. I greet them all by name. "Hey Nurse Faye, Victoria, Eileen, Mary Kate . . . where's Dr. Catevenis?"

It seems like the entire ICU staff on my floor—doctors, nurses, physical therapists, respiratory therapists, medical school students, interns, security guards, nutritionists, maintenance workers—have all rushed into my room. They all want to witness the miracle. I greet as many as I can by name. Everyone looks to be in a state of shock. I'm the only one talking for a change. Not a torrent of words, but enough to cause many to start crying. It's like they have witnessed a corpse climb out of his grave. I owe my life to these people.

The big man, Dr. Catevenis, joins the crowd. I say "hello" again. He then turns around and begins waving his arms as if he is directing traffic. I glance up at the clock; it is 11:00. Visiting hour.

My dad threads his way through everyone. He rushes to my bed to see what is going on.

"Hey Dad! Where's Mom?" He looks at me, speechless, and tears start running down his cheeks. He wants to say something but he is too choked up. I'm the one who has the words now. "Dad, I promise everything is going to be fine."

My mom enters the room. "Hi Mom!" I say. She has the same reaction as my dad, astounded and tearful.

She tenderly places her hand over my right hand. "Hello handsome," she answers.

CHAPTER 12

QUESTION TIME

Now that I can finally converse, it feels like a jailbreak for my mind. Newly freed, I'm determined to ask questions that have circled in my mind like birds of prey hunting for food. Number one priority is finding out why I am here. I keep hearing those two words "car accident," but I have no recollection of being in one. I drive a black 1994 Camaro that I bought from my mom for $2,500. It's a vanity muscle car, but its V6 engine wasn't build for speed. I'm a safe and cautious driver, with no arrests, citations, warnings, or even a single speeding ticket. My friends say I drive like a granny. So how could I have been in a crash, and not just some fender bender? I never raced, drove drunk, or did anything that many eighteen-year-olds often do that raises their parents' auto insurance rates. And if I was driving, what happened to the Camaro or the other driver? Were there any passengers with me? What time of day did the accident happen? Why can't I make sense of any of this? What is preventing me from remembering?

Before the morning nurse arrives, I begin rehearsing the battery of questions that I will ask her. I hope she obliges and answers them. All I want is the truth. It's time I find out the facts. Then I reconsider this strategy. She might feel like she has to protect me from knowing too much if the doctors think it might cause agitation and impede my recovery. But my parents will level with me, won't they? So I will wait until visiting hour before I become Perry Mason.

Meanwhile, I fantasize about water. I'm told that I can't have a sip of water until I pass the swallowing test. Swallowing test? I guess they want to see if I can drink under their supervision. I will have to just wait and suffer.

I'm pleased to see that the morning nurse is Victoria. She is tall, around five feet eleven, and has blonde hair that's usually tied up in a ponytail. She has cared for me numerous times and is always smiling. We exchange small talk at long last. She prepares me for the day's first physical therapy session. My blood is taken, IVs reset, gown changed, and hair combed. I find out that I'm no longer on morphine, though I'm still on the ventilator because my lungs are weak.

My main physical therapist, Francine, walks in and is excited to see that I'm able to greet her. She is usually all business. Or maybe she was only like that with me because I couldn't speak.

Both Francine and Victoria lift me from my bed onto the angry chair. The way it's positioned, I can get a closer look at the photos pinned to the wall. In most of them, I'm in a good mood, smiling. Yet I feel discouraged seeing the muscles I had developed over the many years of weight training and competing in sports. There I am getting ready for a race at a local pool, talking with Coach Covey before a track meet, doing one of my bodybuilding bicep poses. There are several pictures of me with my parents that were taken on our trip to Jamaica in June. Photographic evidence of pre-accident Brian is nearly impossible to reconcile with the present. I must have lost over seventy-five pounds. How am I ever going to get back into shape again? Is that even possible, or will I be confined to a wheelchair? The walls start closing in on me again as I feel the dark, looming pressure of the unknown tightening its grip on the future. I look away from the photos. Thankfully, my therapy session is starting.

We begin with the usual routine of lifting legs, squeezing hands, and pushing feet forward. As we go through each set, I tell them—it's so great to talk!—that it hurts my tailbone when I sit for very long in the angry chair. Victoria says that the pain is due to my broken pelvis, which was shattered in the crash. Since I lost a lot of weight, the tailbone is putting additional pressure on nerves in the area that used to have a lot more body-fat support. She finds a small donut-shaped yellow cushion and places it under my butt. Wow! That's so much better. The pain practically disappears and I thank her for the good deed. She walks outside my room to work on my medical records and daily paperwork.

Under Francine's guidance, I lift my right arm ten times. Even with her direct and serious personality, it's clear that she is amazed at how rapidly the recovery has been going. I glance up at the clock, and I see that it's almost eleven. My parents will be here soon. Will I be able to ask them about the accident? I decide to first test the waters with Francine.

"Um, what other bones were broken besides my pelvis?"

She looks confused. "Nobody has told you?" she responds. I continue to stare at her with a blank look, letting her know that I'm clueless. "Well from your medical records and from talking to your nurses and doctors, I don't really think anybody thought you were actually going to make it. I remember a few weeks ago, I would pass your room and when I looked at you, my heart would break, every single time. You looked like you were in so much pain. I see a lot of patients come in here who are in really bad shape, but you looked like you were ready to slip away any minute. Some people who have undergone much less trauma do die, but here you are. I don't want to frighten you, but I feel like I'm talking to a ghost.

"And, as far as your injuries, I know that many of your ribs were broken, both lungs were collapsed. I was told that your heart had shifted to the opposite side of your chest, but it kept beating because you were fit and healthy. You're like Superman to have gone through what you have, or maybe your heart is just made of iron. Whatever it is, your recovery is beyond belief. You had so many surgeries and operations while you were in the coma. Some of your organs, like your spleen and gallbladder, were removed. You had kidney dialysis, life support, and a ventilator keeping you alive."

Yes, I think, I'm still alive.

She adds, "Because your pelvis was badly damaged from the impact of the crash, that's my big concern at the moment. I'm sorry to have to say this, but it will be another miracle if you can walk again. On the bright side, look how far you have come already."

I now know why my parents and everyone kept telling me that I only had a few broken bones. They never mentioned that I was going to be a cripple the rest of my life. All the progress that I have made has just been canceled. Why did I have to ask Francine? I start crying. She tries to console me, but it's too late.

For the rest of our physical therapy session, I remain quiet and sullen. I try to smile and nod every now and then, but it's completely artificial. My spirit is broken. I'm damaged goods. What will it be like to never walk again? How will this change my life? When I graduated high school a few months ago, I never thought that the bright future I had planned was going to turn into something as awful as this. The day of my graduation, as I walked across the stage, the school principal should have said, "Mr.

Boyle, congratulations, here's your diploma. And by the way, in several weeks, all your goals and dreams will be destroyed in a car accident. Best of luck to you in the future."

When Francine leaves, I'm in a foul mood and I do something that I shouldn't. A white sheet covers me from the waist down. Naturally, I'm curious to see what the rest of my body looks like. From seeing my arms and legs, I know I'm rail thin and have agonizingly come to accept this unfortunate fact. But what does my stomach look like and what about everything below that? I slowly raise the sheet and lift up my hospital gown for a peek. I notice the invading catheter, but as I raise my eyes upward to my stomach and lower chest, the view is revolting. It's much worse than anything I had ever imagined. I have never seen anything as dreadful as this. I knew I was pretty messed up from the accident, but this is totally gruesome. It looks as though I have been ripped open many times by the assistance of scalpels and finely sharpened blades. The only thing missing is the carved signature from the surgeon who did all this fine work. What detail, what craftsmanship. I have scars all over. My stomach has been sliced open from the middle of my chest all the way down to my belly button, and the wound is ugly and red. There are even tiny segments of the skin that have not yet fully closed, and I can actually see tiny holes that go deep beneath the layers of skin. I have another long cut that goes all the way across the lower area of my left pectoral. My body is ruined.

Ever since middle school, I always tried to take care of my physique by eating well and weight training. It started when I joined the basketball team in sixth grade. Every day after practice, I would jump rope for several minutes, do an endless number of sit-ups and push-ups, and run whenever I got the chance.

When I saw the formation of my very first abdominal muscles, the workout craze really hit strong and I weight trained everyday after that. It wasn't really a macho kind of thing that led me to this lifestyle, but more a feeling of being healthy that made me enjoy doing it. The feedback that I happily received from the girls was a big plus too.

Throughout high school, I stayed in shape and actively participated in sports, never getting caught up in the party scene. Shortly after graduation, one of my close friends, named Rachel, persuaded me to pursue modeling. She has the look—tall, blonde hair, long legs, cute face, and she had been modeling for several years. She said that I was the type of guy some agencies were looking for. Shortly after graduation, I received a phone call from a modeling agent in California who wanted me to fly out and attend college near L.A. because he thought I could get work with Calvin Klein Underwear and Abercrombie & Fitch. Unfortunately, I never made the trip west. Instead, I'm in Intensive Care, morbidly staring at my wretched, gone-to-hell body.

When Victoria returns, I hurry to lower the sheet in embarrassment. I give her a fake grin. My parents are following closely behind her, and my dad is carrying a bottle of Mountain Dew. I'm eager to see them. It's a timely diversion from thinking about my Frankenstein torso.

Victoria says that they have a surprise. I can have my first drink. She hands me a small red plastic cup of ice and gives me instructions. I can chew ice but I should let the ice melt so that my mouth will eventually create a swallowing reflex. If I'm able to accomplish this, then I can move onto a sip of water.

I look at the red cup in my hands. I've dreamt of this moment. I bring the cup closer to my lips and feel the cool vapors rising up and caressing my chin, mouth, and cheeks. I can't wait any longer. I slowly bring the cup up, letting the small chips of ice slide into my mouth. My teeth instantly feel a sharp tingling sensitivity to the coldness, but I slowly adjust to it as I swish the ice around my mouth with my tongue. After several seconds, the ice starts to break down into a cold liquid. I feel the tiny muscles in my throat cooperate as the liquid slides down my dry, sandpapery throat. I feel the chill in my stomach. I take another mouthful of ice, a little more this time.

Victoria hands me another red cup, but this one is half-full of water. She repeats the instructions—allow the water to float in my mouth until I feel the need to swallow it. I bring the cup to my lips, pour some of the clear, delicious substance into my mouth, then swallow it. Gaining confidence, I swig down the rest of it in a quick frenzy.

I'm now lusting for some Mountain Dew. My dad seeks permission from Victoria. She nods yes. He unscrews the top and places the plastic bottle in my hands. Without even thinking about how this would be any different from water, I gulp down the Dew. Instantly, I feel an intense burning sensation in my mouth as if I've just drunk a cup of sulfuric acid. That hurts! The burning travels all the way down to my fragile stomach, where it's bubbling. Even with all this discomfort, I continue to drink the painful nectar until the bottle is nearly empty. Oh man, that was delicious in its own crazy way.

The next test is eating Jell-O. Victoria tells me to do the same thing I did with the ice, but instead of just letting it dissolve in my mouth, I should try to chew it up into small slimy fragments. I dip my spoon into the gelatin and scoop out a small amount as if I am digging for gold. I bring it to my mouth and cautiously bite up and down. I don't know if it's really doing anything, but I can tell that it has changed its form in my mouth. I nervously swallow, feeling the soft gooey clumps slide down into my stomach, mixing with the fizzing Mountain Dew. Victoria and my parents start clapping. They tell me that I did a good job. I have just passed my swallowing test with flying colors. I've taken another small step into reentering the realm of normalcy.

From now on, I will no longer receive nutrition from the feeding tube in my nose. Instead I will be eating "soft" food, which will be first mixed in a blender before being served. I'll be like a baby bird receiving food that's already mashed up by its mother. Nonetheless, I'm thrilled, because anything is better than being fed through a tube in your nose. The only bad news is that the feeding tube must be taken out. And yes, Victoria tells me, without anesthesia.

Victoria leaves the room, and I'm alone with my parents. My mom opens up the window blinds behind my bed to let in sunlight. *Ellen* is on. I go back and forth between watching the show and demonstrating to them the progress that I have made with my physical therapy: lifting legs and right arm, wiggling fingers, pushing my feet forward and backward.

They seem happy, content watching me. Then selfishly, I drop the bombshell.

"Exactly just what happened to me?"

They are startled by my question. Mom shoots a nervous glance toward Dad to gauge his reaction. He pauses for several moments, then says in a measured, cautious voice, "Well, son. You were in a really bad car accident."

"Yeah I know that, but what *really* happened? I want to know how and where the accident took place. Was I driving? Did I have any passengers? I'm just trying to understand how I got here, that's all. The last thing I remember is being at your company picnic."

My dad studies the machines keeping me alive. He tells me the police told them that the accident happened around one thirty in the afternoon on July 6, which was three days after the picnic. It took place at an intersection a few minutes from our house at Ripley and Poorhouse roads. I had called them earlier that day because I had just left the track and was on my way to swim at the Lackey High School pool. I mentioned that after my swim workout, I was coming home to lift weights. Then on my way home, I went through the intersection and a dump truck hit me.

"A dump truck?" I ask.

"Yeah," he responds. "The police called it a T-bone because it hit right in the middle of the Camaro on the driver's side."

"And what kind of condition did the police say that I was in?"

My father pauses. It's obvious that he doesn't want to continue. My mom starts talking. She says I called her at work that morning and asked her not to forget to stop by St. Mary's College to make a change to my fall schedule. On her way home, she remembered slamming on her brakes when the car in front of her abruptly stopped as a small dog darted in front of it. For some reason, she looked at the clock and saw the time was 1:30 p.m. She had a strange feeling, almost a premonition. "I often wonder if it was the mother instinct deep within warning me that you were in trouble. It was a feeling that I have never experienced and one I will never forget," she says. Then she stopped at the florist to order flowers for a colleague at work who was in the hospital. She got home around three. As she pulled into the driveway, she noticed that I was still out. Inside, she checked the phone's caller ID and noticed Dimensions Healthcare. She didn't recognize the name and played a message that said, "This is Prince George's Hospital Center calling regarding Brian Boyle. Please call as soon as possible."

"I started trembling, hyperventilating, and crying all at the same time," she says, "I had to dial the number several times because my fingers were shaking so badly. I kept saying to myself, 'What happened? Why Prince George's Hospital?' That's where someone is taken for emergency trauma. When I finally dialed the number, a woman told me that you were in an accident and that I needed to get there soon. I asked over and over if you were alive, but couldn't get any details. The woman asked me if I had someone to drive me there. She could tell that I was frantic. As soon as I hung up, I called your dad on a construction site two hours away. As soon as he answered, I said something bad had happened to you. He screamed into the phone, 'No, No, No! Get to the hospital as soon as you can!'"

My mom stops talking. The memory of July 6 overwhelms her. She can't find the words to carry on. My dad consoles her with a hug. He explains his immediate reaction when he got the bad news. "When I got a call from your mom, I found myself on my knees, like someone had taken a baseball bat and laid me out flat. She told me what hospital and I asked myself if you would be alive when I got there. On my way to the hospital, a police officer from the accident scene called and told me that you were in really bad shape. He said that you had severe internal and head injuries, and he didn't think you were going to survive and was surprised you were still living after the impact of the crash. It was a direct and harsh conversation. The officer didn't show any compassion or empathy."

My dad goes silent.

"How bad did I look when you first saw me?" I ask.

"Son, I know you have a lot of questions about what happened," my dad responds in a shaky voice, "but we aren't ready to talk about that just yet. Everything is still so fresh in our minds right now. Soon, we'll tell you about everything, but we just can't talk about it right now. It's too much."

They sit uncomfortably in their chairs. It seems like we are all lost in our own thoughts. No one says anything for several minutes.

Victoria returns and says it's time to take out the feeding tube, and that it won't be anywhere near as painful as insertion. She gingerly peels back the tape from around the tube in my nose. She places her hands around the end of the tube, prepares me for the moment, and begins tugging.

The tube tickles while coming out. The other end of the thin hollow tube is dripping clear liquid onto my hospital gown. My nose twitches as it regains the feeling of not having a tube jammed in there anymore.

Victoria says that she has more good news. They have been slowly weaning my lungs from the ventilator without my even knowing it. She asks me if I feel any difference with my breathing patterns, and I say no. "Then there is a good chance that the trache tube will be removed."

My parents wait for Victoria to leave before they spring another surprise: Yesterday, between visiting hours, they went to check out two local rehabilitation centers where I can start my real physical therapy.

"You mean . . . I'm going to be leaving here? How soon?" I inquire timidly.

"Yeah, can you believe it?" says my mom. "The doctors said that you have to wait a few days before you can leave because they have to get most of the strong medication out of your system."

"Oh . . . okay, that sounds great. So tell me about the two rehab places."

My dad says, "We visited places in Baltimore and Washington, D.C. Both were highly recommended by the people here. The center in Baltimore is where football players from the Baltimore Ravens usually go when they get injured. We noticed that there was a lot of space outdoors where we could push you around in the wheelchair. The center in Washington was pretty nice too, but we didn't think there was much outside space."

"Okay, yeah, let's go with the center in Baltimore."

Despite only just finding out that I might never walk again, I can't believe everything I'm hearing. My feeding tube is out. I'm finally being weaned off the ventilator. Leaving the ICU is another milestone.

My parents stay for the rest of visiting hour.

RIGHT BEFORE I CLOSE MY EYES FOR A NAP, I NOTICE A FAMILY WALKING by my room, crying and talking quietly with one another. Whoever they are crying for occupies the adjacent room. Both the father and mother are middle-aged. Huddled between them are several teenage-looking boys and girls who, I'm assuming, are their children. One of the older girls is holding up her mom who lifts a tissue to her face, dabbing her red, tearful eyes and then clenching the tissue in her hand the same way my mom used to do. The mother glances in my direction, then averts her eyes and lowers her head because she sees I'm watching. But she raises her head and renews eye contact with me. I smile and raise my right hand to let her know that I understand what she is going through.

She then decides to approach me. Her husband stands by the door. "Excuse me, Brian?" she says in a feeble, uncertain voice. "You don't know me but your nurses told me all about you and everything you went through. Well, my son Brandon is in the same situation that you were in when you first got here." She pauses. "They don't think he is going to make it." Another pause, though much longer, as if she only just realizes the reality of what she has said. "I know you don't know us, but I just wanted to meet you, because everyone keeps telling us that you're a true miracle for making it through all that you have. Just seeing you is giving us all the hope in the world that our son is going to make it, too. Please keep him in your prayers." I tell her that I will. She comes closer to give me a hug. I shake her husband's hand. I tell them to stay strong, and that they should talk to their son as much as they can because he needs them.

When they leave, I easily imagine Brandon in the next room, hooked up to many of the same machines that have kept me alive. I wonder if Brandon is even conscious. Does he know what is going on? Probably not, but one day he will. But what if he doesn't? What if he doesn't make it? I say a prayer for Brandon.

At this moment, I feel like I am the luckiest person in the world to have come this far.

CHAPTER 13

STANDING TALL

A SLEEPLESS, STORM-TOSSED NIGHT. I CAN'T STOP THINKING ABOUT THE costar in my new life: a wheelchair. This new set of wheels will replace the smashed-up Camaro. Hardly a fair trade. No V6 here. Just my hands, arms, and shoulders, which are barely functional. Will I be confined to a motorized chair? I wonder how fast these guys go. I'm sickened by the prospect of being a cripple. And just what is the politically correct term? Handicapped? Paraplegic? Vertically challenged? Disabled? Whatever label society chooses to slap on my forehead, that designation will remain with me the rest of my life. Yes, the rest of my life.

I watch dawn break and the sky lighten from my horizontal perch. I wish it would stay dark and allow me to disappear into its black inky void. I'm not ready for human company. As if to break this moody spell, the physical therapist Francine walks into my room with a metal walker. "What's that?" I ask. "You said yesterday that I was never going to walk again."

"I know I said that," she says with a sly grin, "but I was looking over your X-rays with some of the doctors, and we thought, why not give it a try and see what you are capable of?"

Francine, I say to myself, *you got game!* My mood instantly brightens. "Yes! Let's go for it!" I shout triumphantly.

Another therapist comes into the room, Francine's assistant, holding a belt restraint. They gently slide me over to the left edge of the bed so I can sit upright. My weakened back slouches forward because I'm still getting used to the tug of gravity. Francine's assistant wraps the safety belt around my waist, then puts a pair of socks and shoes on my bony, delicate feet. They slide me forward a few more inches, just enough to regain the sensation of my feet touching the pink-tiled floor. My balance is flimsy. If somebody blew a puff of air at me, I would tip over and shatter into a thousand pieces.

They position the aluminum walker in front of me and move the remaining IVs so they won't get tangled up. The trache tube is unhooked, so from this moment on, I'm breathing entirely on my own. I just hope my lungs are up to the task.

I think back to my power-lifting days, psyching myself up, before I slowly put weight on my feet, ankles, and knees. I tell Francine and her assistant I'm ready. They maintain a sturdy grip on the restraint belt. They lift me. I rise, like Lazarus from the dead. My unused joints make loud cracking noises, like popcorn in the microwave. It takes more than a minute to fully stand. I'm covered in sweat, my back slouching, legs wobbly, arms cramping, lungs heaving. I did it! I stand proudly for another fifteen seconds.

I imagine what it would be like if I took a small step. Just several inches, that's all. But I realize I'm not quite ready for such heroics, so I tell them I need to sit.

They support me as I slowly lean forward, trying to bend my legs. I'm several inches from the bed when my legs collapse and I flop onto the bed—a terrifying but soft landing.

"How did your legs feel?" asks Francine "Did you notice any pain in your pelvis?"

"Nope," I respond enthusiastically. "Just that my legs, knees, and ankles feel so weak. Can we take a break and try it again in a few minutes?"

Francine grants my wish. But just before I try again, my parents arrive. She tells them what we're trying to do. My mother takes out her camera. I feel an intense amount of pressure, but maybe that's what I need right now.

Sitting on the bed, I raise my left foot about two inches off the floor. I do the same with my right leg. I place my hands on the hollow metal rails of the walker, feeling its smooth, cold surface. I take a deep breath, close my eyes, and pull myself off the bed. I stand. All. By. Myself.

My back is as straight as it can possibly be. My scarred chest is held high. I have gone from skeleton boy to Atlas. I grit my teeth and flex what little muscles remain in my forearms and biceps. Heart pounding, I lift my left foot an inch above the floor. I pause in midair and then slide it forward an inch. My first step! Mom snaps a picture and Dad congratulates me, but I'm not done yet. I have to keep going to make sure that this isn't some fluke. I need to test my physical limits. Francine stands next to me, watching intently, ready to offer help with the restraint belt should I falter.

I lift my right foot in the same careful manner, exhale slowly, and clench my jaw, as I slide it forward two inches this time. Another inch with my left and another inch with my right. I keep going. I am now standing outside my room. This is uncharted territory. I feel like I have just walked across the continent. Nurses see me, I smile, and everyone starts cheering. Dr. Catevenis walks toward me, smiling. But after a minute or so, the temporary adrenaline rush fades. I discover that I don't have the strength to turn around and make it back to my room. Uh-oh, I didn't plan for this. I'm in big trouble. I start to panic. If I fall, I will probably break more bones. I visualize my body as a watermelon falling, and the fierce impact causing all its soft insides to burst open.

"Francine! Dad! Help!" I yell. They both rush to my side. Francine holds the safety belt tightly as she helps me turn around to make the return trip. The anxiety dissipates when my body hits the bed. Francine reattaches the ventilator. I spend the next several hours in a state of near exhaustion—and sweet exhilaration.

CHAPTER 14

LEAVING INTENSIVE CARE

When the nurse named Faye arrives, I relentlessly ask her if I can be taken on a tour of the hospital. I'm feeling bold and want to see something else beside Room 19. She keeps telling me that I need to rest but she'll think about it.

When my parents show up, I start pleading with Faye to let them push me around in the wheelchair. Faye finally relents, but she says that due to hospital policy, she will have to be my wheelchair pusher since I'm an Intensive Care patient. I thank her and we prepare for our big trip. My parents put a small pillow on the seat of the wheelchair for my tailbone. Faye unhooks the ventilator and IV tubes and peels off the wired electrodes plastered all over my chest. My parents carry me over to the wheelchair and position my feet into its metal holders.

We roll down the corridor of the Intensive Care Unit talking and having a good time, which, I imagine, is not something that normally happens on this floor. I request a visit to the radiology department. We stop at the double doors that lead to the room with all the CAT scan and MRI machines. I wonder if the perfume-scented technician is here. Would she even recognize me in this condition, since I'm now able to

sit upright and talk? After I spend a few moments staring at these closed
doors and recalling the many times that I have been scrutinized by these
mysterious giant machines, we press on down the hallway.

We go through a door that leads to a large waiting room with chairs,
a television, and another hallway that leads outdoors. I can see the bright
blue sky and the leafy green trees through the windows. I mention that
the ultimate trip highlight would be to go outside. Faye agrees, and we
exit through the automatic sliding glass doors. Once we're outside, I
finally feel free. I'm treated to the smell of the warm summer air, a cool
breeze flowing through my hair, the sound of cars driving by. The sun
feels wonderful on my frail arms and legs. I'm ecstatic, and yet I know
that another difficult journey looms once I leave the hospital and start
my physical therapy at Kernan, the Baltimore rehab. The nurses have
stressed that my new rehab sessions won't be as forgiving as what I've
been doing here.

The other difficulty about leaving Intensive Care is that I will be going
from twenty-four-hour personal care to being pretty much on my own in
an unfamiliar environment. Will I have my own nurses? How will I get
around? I still can't climb in and out of bed by myself. I don't have the
strength to push my wheelchair. And what about all the medications I'm
going to need? It's going to be a really tough transition. After spending
more than two months in Prince George's Hospital Center, I know more
about my room in the ICU than my own bedroom at home. There is
a deep, profound connection I've made with Room 19 that I cannot
explain. I've grown accustomed to its off-white walls and pink-tiled floor,
the aqua-cushioned chair on my left and dark blue chair to the right, the
sink on the left, the clock above the doorway, the television in the upper
right-hand corner. I feel safe and protected as long as I'm in Room 19.

We have been outside for maybe twenty minutes when I decide it's time to head back in because my back and tailbone ache from sitting in the wheelchair. My lungs are also growing weak from the thick humidity and heat. Once we are back in my room, I'm not hooked up to the ventilator or given any new IVs.

Dr. Catevenis walks into my room and tells us that I will be brought up to the eighth floor for the night to make sure that I can handle being in a more independent situation. "Your parents will be able to stay with you, and I will be stopping in every now and then to see how you are doing," he says. "Then, in the morning, you will be transferred to Kernan by ambulance."

As soon as Dr. Catevenis leaves, my parents gather all my things and put them in a large bag. All the photos on the bulletin board are carefully taken down. The bag is nearly to the point of exploding with stuffed animals and get-well gifts from family and friends.

The final few hours I spend in Room 19 are pleasantly filled with eating ice cream, watching television, and chatting with nurses who duck in to say hello.

Two male nurses walk into my room with a wheelchair. My parents stand, greeting them with excitement. My dad cautiously scoops me up from my bed as if I am a small child and places me in the wheelchair. My mom gathers up the rest of my stuff and we make our way down the corridor. Before we get too far, I turn my head for one last look at Room 19 and its collection of now-silent medical monitors and machines that nursed me back from the dead.

ONCE I GET SETTLED IN MY NEW ROOM ON THE EIGHTH FLOOR, I DO something really stupid. It must be a mixture of overconfidence and curiosity to discover what I can do on my own because I try to get out of the wheelchair. After fifteen frustrating seconds, I'm standing but can't go anywhere because my feet are trapped behind the wheelchair's footrests. I didn't think about this before standing. There is nowhere to go but back down in the wheelchair or over the footrests with my feet. I hurry to make a decision, and then it happens: I lose my balance and fall face forward on the bed.

The faceplant triggers a jolt of pain that shoots from my nose all the way down to my toes. It feels as if I have just jumped off a two-story building. My mom rushes over, but my thin legs and feet remain stuck behind the footrests. I can't think straight because the pain is so intense, especially in my legs. I begin to scream. Several nurses rush in my room to help untangle me. My dad, who had been on the Intensive Care floor packing up the rest of my stuff, finally arrives. He pushes the wheelchair out from under me and flips me over on my back. Because my blood pressure is skyrocketing, nurses inject me with several different medications.

I HAVE MY FIRST WHOLE MEAL FOR DINNER: A BIG GREASY CHEESEBURGER with fries and a root beer from a nearby fast-food joint called Five Guys. I then have some ice cream while I watch television with my parents. After an hour, I realize that they are asleep and I slip on my headphones and listen to some of my favorite CDs like *Grassroots* by 311, *What's the Story Morning Glory?* by Oasis, *Stone Blue* by Foghat, *Dr. Feelgood* by Mötley Crüe, and *Powerage* by AC/DC. The music is therapeutic, allowing me to drift off into another world. I stay in this relaxing state until dawn. In just a few hours, I will be moved to Kernan Rehabilitation Center.

CHAPTER 15

KERNAN REHABILITATION CENTER

I have a bowl of cereal for breakfast. Soon afterward, two paramedics enter my room, one pushing a gurney. They put me on it and strap me in tight. My parents walk alongside me as the paramedics push through the hallways and out through the doors of the hospital. An ambulance waits in the driveway. The next time I return to Prince George's Hospital, I want to walk into Intensive Care on my own and personally thank everyone who played a role in my recovery.

The short ambulance ride from Prince George's Hospital to the Kernan Rehabilitation Center seems endless. My dad follows behind in his red Ford F-150 pickup truck. When we arrive at Kernan, the ambulance stops and the paramedics open the rear doors and carefully lift my gurney out of the vehicle and wheel it onto the sidewalk. The sun feels good. The paramedics push me toward the main entrance of the big brick building.

The reception area is filled with nurses and hospital staff, handling paperwork and filling various medications. Several minutes pass before our presence is acknowledged. I wonder if they even knew we are supposed to be here.

After I'm signed in, one nurse who seems friendly leads us down a corridor to my room. But when we take a turn down a hallway with a sign that says SPINAL CORD INJURY UNIT, I'm surprised because I don't have any spinal injuries. My parents are also confused by this and ask the nurse, but she isn't sure why either.

We arrive at my room, which has two beds. The nurse says my roommate was released the previous day. Out of curiosity, I ask about the extent of his injuries. He was a laborer at a construction site when a one-ton block of concrete fell on him and crushed his legs.

The paramedics transfer me to the bed by the windows on the left side of the room. My parents and I thank the men and say goodbye.

The room is plain as vanilla. There are two chairs in the small space between the beds, a television above the door, and a private bathroom on my right.

It takes an hour to settle in. The nurse stops by and tells us that her shift has ended. In a little while, the new nurse arrives. He's unfriendly, less cordial, direct. My parents ask him if they can stay with me overnight because I can't do anything on my own just yet. He declines their request because visitors are not allowed to stay after 9:00 p.m. This is awful. I can't walk or move around without being helped. How will I go to the bathroom by myself? What happens if I have difficulty breathing? Suddenly, I yearn to be back in Room 19, having lunch and talking with the nurses who had become close friends. Perhaps the transition from twenty-four-hour care is too abrupt. Am I really ready to take this next step on the road to recovery?

Because my parents won't budge, Mr. Nurse finally relents. Only one can stay overnight; the other will have to say in a nearby motel. He then checks my vital signs and collects some blood for sampling and tests.

I have been here for less than two hours and I'm already getting stabbed with needles. He leaves with my blood sample but soon returns with a wheelchair, which means escape. I already feel claustrophobic. I ask my parents to wheel me outside, and they are only too happy to oblige.

I sit in the sun and it feels good. The slight summer breeze seems about right for my delicate lungs. Listening to the birds in the trees and cars rush by makes me feel like a normal human being rather than a hospital patient. All I need is a sleeping bag and I'd be content to spend the night under the stars. Just before dusk, my parents wheel me back into the building and down the long hallways to my room.

After a light dinner and an ice cream cone, we watch television and talk about what the first session of physical therapy will be like. There's a knock on the door and a boy, in his mid-teens, arrives by himself in a wheelchair and asks to come in. Sure, we tell him. He rolls right in, like an old friend.

"Hey man, what's up?" he says. "My name is Tony. I heard that you just arrived here a few hours ago. What's your name?"

"Nice to meet you Tony; my name is Brian. Yeah, my parents and I just got here."

Tony says that he's fifteen years old and has been here several months because he is paralyzed from the waist down. He was one of the best football players for his age in the state of Maryland. But during summer vacation he was racing off-road four-wheelers with his buddies when he lost control of the vehicle at fifty miles per hour and collided with a steel guardrail. His neck took the initial impact and his body then wrapped around the metal barrier.

His story leaves me speechless. I feel a strong connection with him. Like me, he's obviously a fighter. But the difference between us is something that I dare not voice: there's a possibility I will be able to walk on my own, while he will be wheelchair-bound for the rest of his life.

Tony's nurse tracks him down in my room and tells him he has to go. Time to take his pain medication. We say goodbye, and I wonder how many patients like Tony are at Kernan—struck down in their youth, with all their hopes and dreams shattered in a split second.

I'm sleepy and my parents let me drift off. Several hours pass before a nurse wakes me, wanting a blood sample. When I awaken again, the morning sunlight is shining through the windows. I have cereal and orange juice for breakfast. My mom decides that for my first session of physical therapy, I should wear something special. She selects a pair of blue shorts and a white T-shirt with the U.S. Naval Academy insignia. Just putting on these clothes leaves me winded.

To get motivated, I listen to various heavy-metal songs on my CD player, with emphasis on the *heavy*—"Awake" by Godsmack, "One" by Metallica, and "Walk" by Pantera. A woman comes into my room. She's tall with blonde hair. "Hello, my name is Karen, and I'll be your physical therapist," she says. We shake hands. My god, her grip is strong.

She wheels me down the long hallway; I attempt small talk but I can tell that she is all business. We take a turn through a set of double doors and I'm wheeled into a large room crowded with other patients. I feel like the new kid on his first day of school. She pushes me a few feet past the door and tells me to wait here because she needs to retrieve my medical file.

I sit alone. Almost everyone here is confined to a wheelchair, both the manual and motorized kind. Several patients are hobbling about using crutches, walkers, or canes. I imagine the age range starts in the teens and reaches into the eighties. Some look like they could be war vets from Iraq, Vietnam, maybe even World War II. I wonder how many are victims of an automobile accident like myself.

Several people are missing an arm or a leg. Some are lying flat on their backs on padded mats, missing all four limbs. In one corner is a small group of patients with heads caved in, eyes missing, and faces half-gone. A teenage boy is sitting in a wheelchair about fifteen feet from me. His head is completely encased by a wire frame bolted into his skull. A trache tube is connected to his life support machine that sits on a nearby cart. His face is rigid and expressionless, with drool spilling down his chin. I too looked this way only several weeks ago.

If I had visited this house of horrors before my accident, I would have been frightened witless. Yet when I peer down at my scarred, shrunken body, I realize that I'm just like all the other unfortunates in this room. I know what it's like to be stared at and judged. How can I ever erase that memory of the young girl who told her mom that I looked like "a monster." Her words cut deeper than a surgeon's scalpel. I still feel the wound.

As I look around at everyone, a fraternity of fellow sufferers, I notice that some are smiling and waving at me. I return their welcoming gestures, feeling an immediate acceptance. One wheelchair-bound man in his late forties is talking to an older woman who must be his therapist. He keeps looking in my direction, and as he shakes her hand to say goodbye, he wheels himself over to where I'm sitting. "Hey buddy, how are you? My name is Gerry. Is this your first day here?" he asks, while extending his hand for me to shake.

"Yes, I just got here yesterday," I respond. "I was in a car accident earlier this summer and just got out of ICU. So how long have you been here?" Behind his grin, there is an overwhelming sadness in his eyes.

Gerry says that he has been here for three weeks because the doctors are trying to see if they can teach him to walk again. When he first arrived, he was technically paralyzed, but his doctors are trying some kind of new therapy to repair his broken vertebrae. I ask him how he broke his back.

His voice turns shaky as he replays the fateful day. "I was a passenger in my brother's car," he says. "We were on the highway. Our mother was sitting in the front seat and my wife was next to me in the back. Our daughter was in between us. A semitruck driving on the left side lost control and rammed into us, killing my brother and mother on impact. My wife and daughter later died in the hospital. I was the only survivor."

I look at him without saying anything. Tears roll down his cheeks. I reach out my hand to him, holding onto his shoulder and offering sympathy as I get choked up as well.

Listening to Gerry and then thinking about paralyzed-for-life Tony, I understand that everyone here has an equally painful and tragic story. Including me. One day, you are fine. Driving home from swim practice, dune bugging with your pals, or traveling somewhere with your family, and then *bam*, out of nowhere, your life is changed in an instant and you find yourself living in a different world. You only hope that with the promise of rehab to mend your damaged body, your spirit won't break as well.

Karen comes back and says in her drill-sergeant voice, "Let's get to work." As she wheels me away from Gerry, I tell him to stay strong. He gives me a brave smile in response. We pause at an empty area in the center of the room. She drapes a heart rate monitor around my neck.

It has a wire cord that she attaches to my right index finger. My blood pressure is alarmingly high, she notes. She wheels me over to a wood-framed mattress and helps me onto a blue padded mat. She asks me to raise one leg and then the other and to do the same with my arms. While I'm doing these movements, she measures my flexibility. After she records the results, she helps me get back into the wheelchair and pushes me over to a table.

"Your blood pressure is way too high," she says with a hint of sarcasm. "You really have to just relax. This is a big concern, so I think this will be about as much stretching that I'd like to do with you today in your first session. Your body just needs time to adjust. We don't want you having a stroke in here."

She then hands me a small piece of plastic with wheels. It looks like a child's toy. What am I supposed to do with this object? She tells me to push it forward and backward on a table. I'm able do it with my right hand, but due to the severe nerve damage in my left shoulder, my left hand can only budge it several inches. It feels so damn weird not to have strength in my left arm, but that's how it is. Karen reassures me that I might one day have full recovery with my left shoulder and arm but it will take two to three years. I had heard that same prognosis from nurses back in Intensive Care. I just have to be patient. Do I have any other choice?

After my first session of physical therapy, Karen wheels me back to my room. My parents are waiting. We have a small lunch and then we go outside and take a tour of the grounds.

Something has been troubling me for several days, and as much as I hate to disrupt the tranquil mood as my parents roll me down the pathways, I can't resist the temptation. I say to my dad, "You never finished telling me what happened when you first arrived at the hospital."

He looks at me with surprise. So does my mom. But they realize that they can't put off revealing the facts anymore. He wheels me over to some shade underneath a tree. They both take a seat on a nearby concrete bench. He begins: "When I finally got to the hospital, which seemed like it took forever, I walked into the waiting room and saw your mom, Uncle Pat, Aunt Donna, and Uncle Joe, who had all already arrived. A receptionist told me that you had just come out of surgery and were in the recovery room and a nurse took us there. The situation was unreal. There were doctors and nurses gathered all around you. Machines were plugged into your body, with tubes running everywhere, including a big blue cylinder-type breathing tube in your mouth. There was a fresh, ugly red surgical cut running from your belly button up to your chest.

"I said, 'Brian, Mom and Dad are here. We love you, son; you're going to be all right buddy. Don't give up.' After I said that, your body started to thrash around, but you were not conscious. As the nurses tried to hold you down, I thought to myself, 'This can't be happening.' I asked the nurses if you would survive and their only response was that you were now in God's hands. Then it was time for us to leave. We stopped in a stairwell and your mom wept. A little later in the waiting room, a nurse arrived and asked us to follow her. She offered no details. 'I just need you to come with me,' she said. We walked in silence. We thought we were on our way to the morgue. The elevator door opened, and we followed her down a short hallway to another set of doors. We had no idea where she was leading us."

My dad pauses; the memory of that first day is tough to relive. "We were taken to Room 19, which was right in front of the nurses' station because they wanted to keep close tabs on you." He says that I was sedated and unconscious, surrounded by more nurses and doctors, more machines and more tubes. There were so many things going on that they couldn't even come close to touch me.

He tells me it was gut-wrenching. "It was the first time as parents that there was not a thing that we could do for you. You already looked like you were dead."

When I hear that word, "dead," I almost don't want to know what comes next. But he says that they stumbled back to the waiting room, unable to describe what they had seen to the others. They were in a state of shock. Everyone left for the night, but they stayed in the waiting room. My dad was still in his work clothes, with concrete chips in his hair. They couldn't leave. A little while later, a physician's assistant by the name of Mary Kate came over to speak with them. She was a serious professional medical person who had seen everything during her career. She said that she needed to ask a few questions about me: my age, existing medical conditions, and so on. She asked them if I was their only child. Yes, they said. Tears rolled out of her eyes. Then she left, and they waited, minute-by-minute, hour-by-hour, in silence. There was another woman in the waiting room with them. Her husband had fallen off a ladder while he was working on their home and hit his head.

Dad says that around one in the morning, Dr. Daee walked in. He was the lead surgeon when I arrived at the trauma unit by helicopter. It was their first meeting with him. He tried to be positive without going into extreme details. He then left and they continued sitting there, in quiet disbelief, for the rest of the night while watching the door to the trauma ward, fearing that if it opened, they would hear that I had passed away.

My dad stops talking and I try to find some words to respond to everything I've just heard, but I can only sit with my hands crossed and head bent in silent reflection. My mom tries to lighten the mood by looking at her watch and saying that it's almost time for my next session of therapy, where I will relearn basic skills such as tying a shoe, putting on clothes, using the toilet.

My parents wheel me back to the physical therapy room. It's the first time that they have been in here. I say hello to Gerry, who is working with his therapist.

A new therapist walks over to greet us. Her name is Jamie and she is gorgeous, with blonde hair down to her shoulders. I'm excited to start the session, especially with a beautiful therapist at my side. "I think I'm starting to like this place," I whisper to my parents.

Jamie sits down in a chair next to a table and reviews my medical file. She then asks about my injuries. I explain that I'm having trouble with my tailbone and my left arm. She tells me to lift my left and right arms on command. She proceeds to measure the strength in my hands with a mechanical gripping device that shows output in watts of power. I feel my blood pressure rising, and not just because of the physical exertion. Jamie's beauty is overwhelming.

Next up is measuring the strength of my arm muscles. She wraps the same blood pressure contraption around my neck that I used with Karen and places the analyzing device around my fingertip. She gives me a two-and-a-half-pound dumbbell and asks me to do some bicep curls with my right arm. I look at the weight, thinking it should be easy, but as I start to lift it, my arm feels odd and weak. This is a huge blow to my self-esteem because three months earlier, I was able to curl fifty pounds per arm for repetitions; and now here I am barely able to lift this ridiculously small weight. I try to shrug off my frustration with laughter. I guess Jamie won't be impressed by my weightlifting prowess.

It's time to test my legs. Jamie wheels me over to two waist-high, parallel-to-the-ground metal poles and helps me out of the wheelchair. As I stand up, I feel dizzy and hold onto the poles for support. Meanwhile, Jamie wraps a belt around my waist for added security. My pulse is racing.

I wait until I'm calmer before I take my first step. I concentrate, then put weight on my right foot as I slide it forward a few inches. With Jamie's encouragement, I try the same thing with my left foot, moving it forward another few inches. I repeat with my right foot, then left, and so on. I make my way to the middle of the poles—a distance of five feet—and I am winded. My legs ache with fatigue. Jamie tells me to turn around slowly so I can return to the wheelchair. As I rotate to my left, I see for the first time that there is a full-size mirror next to the parallel poles. In its reflection is a skeletal-looking boy. Who can that be? He's Holocaust survivor–thin. There is no way it's me. I couldn't have lost *that* much weight. I slowly raise my hand to confirm my denial, but the hand in the reflection also raises, just like that mirror scene in the Marx Brothers' *Duck Soup.*

Suddenly, thousands of tiny bright lights explode in my brain and my legs buckle. I start to fall, but Jamie quickly yanks the restraining belt to hold me up and the poles snag my armpits, where I dangle like a useless puppet without its master. As if from a great distance, I hear Jamie shouting for help. Moments later, I pass out.

When I come to, I realize that I'm still in the physical therapy room. Jamie is talking quietly to me, dabbing my forehead with a moist towel. I have no energy except to wanly return her smile. But deep down, I can't escape the grotesque image of seeing myself in the mirror. I lean back against the wheelchair's headrest, letting my head hang loosely as I gaze at the ceiling with my mouth open, making a sick groaning sound. I feel eyes watching me from all around, but I don't care.

My parents arrive and Jamie walks over to greet them, saying that I did surprisingly well and covered a lot of ground. I wonder if Jamie will tell them that I blacked out. She doesn't. Nor will I. My parents look happy. Why spoil their mood?

They wheel me out of the physical therapy room and down the light-colored tile hallways. We turn into a small cafeteria area and buy an ice cream cone to celebrate my first day at rehab even though there were mixed results. I keep quiet about who or what I saw in the mirror. We move outside to a secluded place on the center's grounds and find ourselves by a small pond stocked with koi. This must be a meditation garden where patients and family can seek tranquility, because in this place of wrecked bodies and smashed dreams, that peace is priceless.

Between small bites of chocolate ice cream, I ask my parents who is going to stay with me tonight. My dad says that he will. It's still midafternoon, so we have time to relax. As we watch the colorful fish swim in lazy looping circles, I ask him to continue talking about those first days in Intensive Care. He looks uncomfortable, but after some hesitation, he begins where he last left off. "In the morning, your mom and I were wide-awake in the waiting room, just waiting and waiting. The ICU door finally opened, but the doctor went over to the woman sitting next to us and he asked her to come with him to the adjoining room. Seconds later, we heard her loud cries of pain. We hoped that we would never have to be taken to the 'debriefing room.'"

A nurse named Kay then came out to tell them that I had made it through the night but I was still in very critical condition. They still didn't know the full extent of my injuries. She took them back to Room 19, where once again, I was surrounded by a small swarm of nurses, doctors, machines, feeding tubes, chest tubes, breathing tube, drip bags, a neck brace, canisters filled by drainage tubes. The raw surgical cuts on my chest were oozing bright red specks of blood. Everywhere else on my body were dark purple, almost black bruises and shattered cuts from broken glass. The sight took their breath away. Even though I was unconscious, I started thrashing around. The doctors and nurses tried holding me down while others ran into the room to assist. My parents left the room and watched through the glass window in complete silence. One of the nurses came running out of the room, asking, "What else can we give him? We have given him everything already." When they looked back in the room, one of the doctor's feet were off the ground, and I was pulling him onto the bed with my right arm. As I finally calmed down, they were left in sheer terror at what they had just witnessed.

What they witnessed, I can't recall. Nothing, not the thrashing, not lifting the doctor off the ground with one arm. All of this seems too unbelievable. I wonder what other things Dad saw. I ask him to go on.

Kay told them that if I lived, it would be a roller-coaster ride. So my parents went back to the waiting room where some family and friends had arrived, and once again, they had no words to describe what they had just seen. All they could say was that I was still alive and fighting. My track coach Mr. Covey came and sat with me for quite a while. As things progressively got worse, the nurses said even though I was heavily sedated, the visits were agitating me to the point where they would have to give me more drugs to calm me down. At that point, my parents decided to end the visits. They asked everyone, including the family, to go home. It was a difficult decision to make and they felt bad about it.

"We had no rule book or guidance about how to handle this, or what we were supposed to do," he says. "We met Dr. James Catevenis and Dr. William Boyce, more great men, the head doctors in Intensive Care. We came at them with questions from every angle hoping to get more information about your status, but it always produced the same response. Dr. Catevenis, looking very serious, would always say, 'We'll just have to wait and see.' Sometimes, when Dr. Boyce would see us in the hospital hallway, he would turn and walk the other way to avoid us. Months later, he told us that he felt so bad for us, and there had been no definite answers about whether you would live or die. At the time, the doctors told us that they wanted to place you in a chemically induced coma to keep your body still. A nurse said that it might seem like they were torturing you with all the things they had to do to try to save you. Later that day, Dr. Daee came out and told us he would have to take you back into surgery because of internal bleeding."

I ask my dad how long they stayed at the hospital before they finally went home. He tells me that they finally left the hospital on the third day to go home, clean up, change, and rush back to the hospital. It was hard walking into the house. My mom says, "Your cereal bowl was still on the table from the day of the accident. We went to your room. We sat on your bed, crying, never having felt so lonely in our lives. Home was not our happy place anymore. One of us was missing. It was an empty shell. Our lives completely stopped. Nothing existed in our world but you."

I realize that I should change the subject. "Can we get some more ice cream?" Relieved, my parents wheel me back inside the building to the cafeteria. It's been a long day. I have enough information for now.

CHAPTER 16

WHERE AM I?

faint beeping noises from the machines surrounding me. Why am I on life support and being pumped full of morphine? I'm in a total panic, and with adrenaline soaring, I pull out my bladder catheter. There's a plastic tube going into the left side of my chest. I give it a gentle tug, just to see if it's securely fastened. There's a slight hesitation; it's lodged deep within my body. But with more force, I pull it so hard that I hear a "pop" and it breaks loose; then I rip it out completely. Warm liquid spurts out, covering the bed and my hospital gown in blood. I search around for more tubes and find a thin one going into my nose. I wrap my fingers around the feeding tube and yank hard. It takes forever to pull it out. I grab the electrode wires connected to my arms, chest, stomach, and quickly detach them. I'm possessed with superhuman strength. I grab the blood pressure cuff on my left bicep, tearing off the Velcro strap and hurling it across the room. Then I come to the big round tube that goes into my mouth, I try to pull that one out, but there's an uncomfortable sensation deep within my chest. So I shift focus to the plastic assembly connecting the two tubes through my throat. This is the ventilator and it's routed to the pathways of my respiratory system. I don't know if I can get these two tubes out, but I can't stay in this bed any longer. It's definitely a huge risk, but I grip the right railing and slide my right foot over the edge. If I can get off the bed and onto the floor, maybe the tubes will break free and I can crawl away. I can't stay in this room any longer. If I don't leave now, I don't think I'll ever make it out of here alive. I have to escape. Now is my only chance for freedom.

A nurse walks around the corner and sees me climbing out of the bed. She shouts for help. Soon there are several people grabbing me from all sides, but I fight them off, violently punching and kicking. I have the strength of five men. Machines are knocked over, a bag of intravenous fluid splashes on the floor. I'm being stabbed with needles—painkillers, sedatives, morphine—yet they feel like harmless pinpricks. In a fit of rage, I grab the largest man in the room, Dr. Catevenis, with my right arm and try to lift him up in the air.

Finally, my strength starts to ebb from all the drugs. I release the doctor. His feet find the floor. I soon grow numb and listless, resigned to the fact that I will never leave this room. The medication has foiled my plan. I lie back on the bed, glassy-eyed, defeated. The sheets are drenched in blood, sweat, and a tangle of disconnected medical wires and tubes. Nurses hurry to clean up the mess. They insert the tubes back in the side of my chest, and for safe measure they stitch them into my skin. They reattach the electrodes, heart rate monitor, blood pressure cuff, IVs, feeding tube, and catheter. My arms and legs are strapped down tightly over clean sheets.

The ceiling grows blurry. Industrial-strength painkillers are taking me to a faraway place. In the distance, I hear a familiar voice.

"Brian? Son, are you awake?"

Huh? It takes me a few moments to realize that I just had a bad dream. I'm drenched in sweat. Room 19's ceiling is in fact the ceiling of my Kernan room. It's late afternoon, and the sun's slanted rays fill the room with a soft light. I look over and see my dad sitting up in the bed on the other side of the room. It's a comforting, reassuring sight.

"Are you okay?" he asks.

I groggily nod yes, but as I try to shake off the effects of this naptime nightmare, I'm unsure how much was made up and how much was actually real. Was my memory trying to reconstruct itself from buried fragments? Did I really act that way in Room 19, like a caged beast fighting for its freedom? Will I ever remember what happened during those first few weeks in Intensive Care? Do I even want to go there? Isn't it wiser to keep the past as far away as possible? Or does this mean that I can expect to have many more nightmares as my subconscious attempts to fill in all the missing elements? I can't deny the obvious: any recollection from being in the coma is like a jigsaw puzzle with permanently missing pieces. Suddenly, I feel nauseous and vomit over the side of my bed. The acidic liquid burns as it gushes up through my throat and out my mouth. Red liquid puddles on the tile floor. I hope it's not blood but the remnants from the fruit punch that I drank earlier. My dad hurries to get a towel to clean up the floor. He looks disgusted.

"Come on, Dad, you have to have a stronger stomach than that," I joke, as he swabs up the vomit. He helps me change into a different shirt.

Several hours of daylight remain, so we decide to go outside. He lifts me out of the bed and helps me into the wheelchair. We're soon rolling out the door and down the empty hallways. Every room we pass, I look inside. Most of the patients are alone. No friends, no family. They all look lonely. Then I think about Gerry, who lost his entire family.

We exit the building and say hello to the other patients in their wheelchairs. Tony's wearing a hoodie even in the heat. I give him a high-five greeting.

My dad pushes me along down a new path. We approach a two-story building at the base of a small hill. This is the Traumatic Brain Injury Unit. We peer through the windows. In each room, there are several patients lying next to each other in separate beds. Each vegetative person is hooked up to machines whose digital readouts flash every few seconds. I can faintly hear the machine's beeps, going on and off like a never-ending orchestra in their closed-off world. These patients' chests automatically rise and fall from their ventilators. Their eyes are frozen wide-open. I ask my dad if that was how I looked when I was in a coma. He glumly nods yes.

When I was in Intensive Care, it was assumed that I might end up in the Traumatic Brain Injury Unit, which is the medical dumping ground for those who are neither living nor dead; it's the final resting stop before the cemetery. I can easily see myself lying in one of those beds, my wide-open eyes like blank marbles. I can't help but wonder if their brains are functional enough to allow any kind of thought, or if they have been too severely damaged. Only during the later stages of my coma was I able to regain a partial sense of my surroundings. I shudder to imagine being indefinitely trapped inside a walled-off cocoon, completely cut off from all human interaction. Yet that's what many thought would be my fate. The kid in the coma. Me.

I have to get away from here. It's too much to bear. Just then, a nurse catches us looking into the window, so she closes the blinds to block our view. Rebuked, we move down the path.

As we roll along, I ask Dad what it was like for him and Mom to spend day after day at the hospital, how they coped with the waiting, what they did.

He tells me that every day for two months, they did the same thing: woke up early, got to the hospital. Visiting hours were limited in ICU. They were allowed three one-hour visits daily, at 11:00 a.m., 2:00 p.m., and 5:00 p.m., which were not enough. They'd stay all day and leave at eight o'clock. On most nights, they drove home in silence, neither wanting to talk about whether I was going to live. Every night at eleven o'clock and every morning at seven, they got a call from a nurse to give them my status. The hardest part was constantly hearing that "I was in God's hands." My medical updates were always dismal. Things seemed to get worse as time went on. Every day there was something new, something worse.

I was never in a full-body cast for my broken bones. My parents asked the doctors why and were told that it was not a priority because my insides were so massacred. Too much internal injury had to be taken care of first.

My dad pauses and says, "You might not like to hear all this."

"I need to know. I really do."

"Here goes . . . "

The list is endless; severe concussion; serious heart complications due to its having been jolted out of its normal position—it had moved several inches across my chest; my heart sac filled with blood; torn diaphragm; collapsed lungs; spleen removed; lacerated liver; kidney dialysis; bowels and intestines squeezed upward due to the sheer impact of the accident. My father tells me that he learned from one of the policeman at the accident scene that there was less than five inches of space between the car door and the front console; my shattered pelvis was compressed into that small space. The doctors said it was like a water balloon being squeezed, causing my bowels and intestines to shoot up through my body. There wasn't an organ in my body in the right place, and every one was damaged or bruised. I had broken ribs and a broken clavicle, and possible spine and brain injuries. One day, as the nurses worked on me, the bed covers came off, exposing my naked body. My parents noticed that my testicles were the size of grapefruits and black as coal. This really freaked them out, but they were told that it was a symptom associated with severe blunt-force trauma in men.

I look at my dad, feeling embarrassed. But he continues.

"One surgeon by the name of Dr. Nafisy explained to us that when you were first brought into surgery and Dr. Daee cut open your chest, he had to lift up your heart and move it across your chest. Usually, Dr. Nafisy said, most hearts would have stopped, but yours kept beating."

These details sweep over me like a tidal wave. I ask him how much blood I lost.

He tells me that by the time I arrived at the trauma unit by helicopter forty-five minutes after the accident, I had already lost about 60 percent of my total blood. I needed thirty-six blood transfusions and thirteen plasma treatments in Intensive Care.

I never knew I was that close to death. But there's one more thing I want to find out—at least now. "Dad, did my heart ever give out in surgery or any other time?"

He doesn't say anything for several minutes. I know it must be hard for him. Finally, he says, "To this day, your mom and I still don't know all the specifics. Some of the nurses told us that your heart stopped seven or eight times during those two months in ICU. We never asked for more details, because frankly we just didn't want to find out."

CHAPTER 17

THERAPY SESSIONS

I HAVE SETTLED INTO A REGULAR ROUTINE AT KERNAN. EVERY MORNING, a nurse wakes me up at six o'clock to take some blood. I eat breakfast at eight, and my first bout of physical therapy with Karen starts at noon.

Her stern, drill-sergeant approach starts with a random selection of arm and leg raises. If my blood pressure and pulse are high, we switch to something easier. On the third day, she isn't available, so I work with Derrick, an older man who's even more aggressive and direct than Karen. He makes me stand on each leg for several seconds to improve my balance. But with my weak muscles, I wobble briefly on my left foot, then nearly fall flat on my face. Luckily, he catches me in time.

As I continue the balancing exercise while holding onto a wall for support, Derrick asks about my sports background. I mention I was on my high school swim team and that I've been thinking about getting back in the pool—especially since I found out that the center has an indoor pool. He shakes his head and tells me swimming is unlikely due to all my injuries. "I'm sure you have a lot of fight in you, kid," he says. "You're definitely a survivor, but this is reality we're talking about. I have looked over your medical file, and it says that you were on life support for two months. Hell, man, you're an animal and there's no doubt about it. But getting back in the pool with the way your body is now, I just don't think it's likely. You're living, you're walking—you've got a future ahead of you. You'll find something else besides swimming, I can promise you that."

I complete the therapy session in silence, keeping my anger over his remarks in check. I have a strong inkling that there will be plenty more naysayers like Derrick in my new life, telling me what I *can't do* rather than what I *can do.*

I look forward to my 3:00 p.m. occupational therapy session with the beautiful Jamie. If she only knew what a hopeless schoolboy crush I have on her. She's hot, several years older, and look at me—I'm just a pathetic bag of skin of bones. What attractive girl would want to spend time with a banged-up guy like me? Yet Jamie is sensitive, tender, caring; she makes me feel like a normal person. I wonder if she's always this nice and sweet with her patients. She is a saint.

Jamie's job is to teach me how to do simple everyday chores. We start with tying shoelaces. She places a black Nike running shoe on the table in front of me. I stare at it. Nothing really intimidating, right? But looks are deceiving, because my left hand refuses to cooperate with my right. I flop my left hand upon the shoe for support as I ready my right hand to do all the work. You would think that I'm a diamond cutter by the intensity I direct toward this simple act. I take a break after the first loop. Several minutes later, I have the next loop established. My fingers fumble trying to interweave the loops for a knot. After fifteen minutes, I finish tying my first shoelace.

When Jamie shows me how to take a sponge bath in the middle of the therapy room without water, soap, or sponge, I'm self-conscious and red-faced. My pulse is quickened, but it's not from panic or fear; I'm sure of that. As she guides my hands through the motions of what it will require to take a bath, my imagination is running wild. I see us in a bathtub together. My scars have healed. I have gained back all my weight and muscles. She rubs shampoo into my scalp. I feel her soft breasts against my broad back. She leans forward and places a dollop of soapy foam on my nose and lets out a sexy laugh. I splash water at her in response. She hugs me tight—so tight I want to burst with passion.

Oh well. A guy can have his fantasies; no harm with fun make-believe, especially in a place like this. That's the cruel joke about rehab: almost everyone initially thinks that things will eventually return to the way they used to be. But that's misguided and wrong; there's a distinctive before and after. Some things will never be the same again.

I look around this room and see people just like me struggling to perform the most basic, minimal tasks in front of their therapists. Full-grown men cry out in pain as they try to bench-press a broomstick. A young boy struggles to learn how to walk after a drunk driver ran him over. A young girl hides her tears behind sunglasses. She lost her arms and legs to a flesh-eating disease. She can't be more than twelve years old. She has brown hair that falls to her shoulders and is neatly tied in the back with a yellow ribbon. She wears a tank top. All four limbs are now stubs, so she must learn how to sit up in a chair without falling over.

It's all here, the breathtaking sadness, the human misery. But when you take away the catastrophic injuries, you find regular people who once lived normal everyday lives.

A young, muscle-bound guy, probably in his late twenties, looks like he recently fought in Iraq or Afghanistan because he is wearing a U.S. Marines T-shirt and has a military haircut. A large white bandage is wrapped around his waist. He sits quietly in a chair, while his therapist continually checks his bandages for seepage.

Surprisingly, the older women in this room, most of them in wheelchairs—probably due to broken hips from falls—are the most active, often doing flexibility exercises with their arms.

Single-leg amputees learn how to use a cane or a crutch. The double-leg amputees are usually on the soft blue mats spread out on the floor, their freshly amputated limbs covered in white gauze.

There is a limited degree of competition between everyone, but the real rivalry is not with one another. Instead, the challenge remains an internal battle, conducted entirely within our own private hell. Victory is measured in the smallest achievable increments. Like tying a shoelace.

CHAPTER 18

WITNESS

STROLLING THROUGH THE CENTER'S SPRAWLING GROUNDS WITH MY parents, I continue to press them for more details about Intensive Care. Because my memory is an incomplete, smudged blur, I believe that for my rehab to be ultimately successful, I need to know more about what happened to my body.

From what my dad has already said, my body was the site of a medical war fought minute-by-minute, hour-by-hour, day-by-day. The battlegrounds were my displaced and smashed up heart, lungs, kidneys, liver, bladder, spleen, gall bladder, bowels, intestines, stomach, brain, bones, and my blood loss.

"The complications were endless," Dad emphasizes. "It seemed like we were signing authorization papers for surgeries every other day. Each time was more heartbreaking. You made it through the first week, which surprised everyone, even us. But things didn't get better; they got worse. More surgeries, blood clots, blood transfusions. You needed a tracheotomy to continue breathing on life support. The breathing tube through your mouth could only be used for a short time because of the chance of infection."

Dad tells me that the breathing tube was placed in my neck with a huge tubular cylinder, which looked like a vacuum hose and was attached to a big machine with a monitor. The tube had a plug with a slender plastic tube feeding into a canister. This was done to suction out my lungs. He tells me the canister would fill up constantly with what looked like chunks of raw meat. This last detail is gross. But this was my daily reality, a constant clashing between infection setting in and medical technology hoping to curb it. But medicine was losing.

Pneumonia, infections, and fever set in on top of everything else. Then came the dreadful day came when the trache tube clogged up and I turned blue from lack of oxygen. My parents had seen me for the morning visit and were sitting out in the front lobby to wait until the two o'clock visit. About an hour later, a nurse asked them to come with her and see Dr. Catevenis. Once again they thought this was it, and they literally ran down the halls. When they got to my room, everyone looked disheveled; Dr. Catevenis was sweating, and nurses were everywhere. I looked like a body lying in a morgue. Dr. Catevenis said to them, "I think I got to him in time."

"They weren't sure how many minutes your brain had gone without oxygen," says Dad. "Then Dr. Daee came in and Mom was crying. He hugged her and told us they were going to take you back into surgery to insert a new vacuum tube for your breathing."

Then he tells me that the doctors were forced to chemically paralyze me to help heal my damaged insides. They came in to see me and I looked like death. My blue eyes looked almost black. No sign of life. "We were so numb at this point, but we couldn't give up on you. There was something deep inside you fighting to live," he says.

I was put into a bed that looked like something out of a science fiction movie. It had compartments to fit my torso, head, legs, and arms. Once I was secured with straps, the bed tilted to from side to side to keep my body in motion so my lungs wouldn't fill up with fluids.

I learn that they kept me in this special bed contraption for five days because the paralysis medicine was so strong it could damage the brain. After I was returned to my regular bed, they started to wean me off the heavy medicine and placed me back in the chemical coma. Then, another kind of bed was brought in. "This one swayed you from side to side," Dad says. "But your infections were getting worse, and the doctors were trying to pinpoint what they were and where they were coming from; they suspected either the gall bladder or liver. After more tests were conducted, Dr. Daee said that you needed an operation to remove the gall bladder. He informed us that he 'doesn't like to cut unless absolutely necessary,' but we knew surgery was inevitable."

As the weeks went by, things looked increasingly bleak. By August, it seemed hopeless, but I was still clinging to life. They were so tired, sad, broken, and lost in a world in which they had no control. My fever continued and infection lingered. The nurses wrapped me with big bags of ice and covered me with a silver ice blanket to try to lower my body temperature. I would shiver intensely from the cold. Then came a jolt of more bad news.

Dr. Saeed Koolaee, the cardiologist, saw that I had fluid around my heart, which was squeezing the organ and building rapidly. The next day, Dr. Daee and Dr. Nafisy, the cardiac surgeon, double-teamed the surgery. Dr. Daee removed my gall bladder and Dr. Nafisy installed a drainage tube to reduce the excess fluid around the heart.

Eventually, the doctors decided to slowly turn down the coma sedation, which was two hundred times stronger than morphine, to see the response. Even though I was chemically unconscious, I would get agitated. Then something happened—a day they never thought would arrive. "You opened your eyes halfway," my dad says. "You stared at us for about ten minutes, and then your eyes closed. There was no movement in any other part of your body, but we would take anything we could get. The doctors continued to slowly wean you off the coma sedation medication. Yet the more awake you became, the more terrified you looked each time you opened your eyes. Just your eyeballs would move as if you were trying to look around the room. That was it. There was no other movement in your body. We couldn't imagine what you were thinking. Mom would massage your face hoping it would trigger some response. Then a fever came back with a vengeance. After several days, you opened your eyes again and closed them about halfway. It seemed like you were trying to blink, letting us know that you were there."

I recall that first blink. Then I began to have those seizures.

My father explained it was from withdrawing from medication. I was a health-conscious kid who never got into drugs, drinking, or smoking. The doctors even told my parents that my blood was spotless of any chemicals—that was rare to see nowadays. Taking me off all the medicine got rough. "You didn't just have a monkey on your back," says my dad. "You had a gorilla." Drug withdrawal is devastating to watch.

My parents had to witness the misery on my face, while my body sweat profusely. I was vomiting all the time, which was scary because I was still on life support and there was the threat of the trache clogging. My body stayed in the fetal position with my knees touching my chin. I shook uncontrollably. "The drugs that saved your life," he says, "now became the demons you had to fight. Then the high fevers struck again. Out came the ice and cooling blankets. Your eyes were open but staring straight out into space."

Yeah, I must have looked like a zombie junkie in detox. But the truth is that the doctors rolled the dice with the heavy drugs, because without them I would have died.

"The first time we saw you strapped into the chair," continues my dad, "we thought that you were brain-damaged. One of the nurses told us this is also called 'death without a funeral.' We were both shocked but couldn't show it. We just stood there in silence asking ourselves, 'When is he going to get better?' You had lost so much weight—just skin and bones. You were slumped sideways, eyes dazed with a blind stare, and your mouth hung open with drool running down your chin. We were willing to deal with whatever it would take to get you back, brain-damaged or not. But the next day, your eyes were open and blinking on command. Later that day, you moved your lips trying to talk but nothing came out. We wanted to think you were saying, 'I can't talk.' This meant a lot to us. It suggested you were aware even in your locked-in state. We had hope again."

On subsequent visits, he says, I showed more positive signs of life. I would blink more. I even nodded slightly when the night nurse asked if I'd like to watch the 2004 Summer Olympics. But two days later, everything seemed to be going in reverse. They walked into my room in the morning to find me staring at the ceiling again. They tried to get a response from me but got nothing. I looked like I was giving up. "As we left your room, we walked through the big double doors of the ICU ward thinking, 'We've come this far. What's happening now?' As Mom started to cry, I told her, 'I think Brian is giving up. He's leaving us now.' She thought the same thing. So on the second visit that day, I started yelling and swearing at you. 'Brian, we need you to fight now; you are the only thing we have in our lives.' I could see fright, panic, terror, exhaustion, and confusion in your eyes."

I can't help but wonder why the fight went out of me then, especially after I had battled for so long. What's remarkable is that my dad wouldn't let me disappear into death's void. His tough-love bedside sermon marked the true beginning of my recovery, because the next day I was able to smile, blink more, even wag a finger. While I had another bad spell for about a week with seizures and tremors, I had definitely turned the corner. But without my parents' support and love, that route could just as easily have become a tragic dead end.

PART TWO

BODY

CHAPTER 19

COMING HOME

I HAVE ONLY BEEN AT KERNAN FIVE DAYS, BUT I'M GOING HOME TODAY. Our health insurance provider decided to cut short the length of my stay because it thought that my rehab could be done at much lower cost through twice-weekly outpatient treatment. I can't wait to leave Kernan even though I'm still in bad shape. I can walk maybe ten to fifteen feet unaided, with someone on the other end of the restraint belt just in case I fall. I can bicep-curl two and a half pounds with my right arm and bench-press a broomstick. But apart from the lovely Jamie, the therapists and nurses are much less friendly than those at Prince George's Hospital where I was treated like royalty. At Kernan, I feel like I'm just another anonymous patient in its body-mending factory about to be spat out into the world as a defective product. I feel sorry for those like Tony who have languished here for months.

My parents are excited as they pack my wheelchair, clothes, walker, and the rest of my belongings in Dad's pickup truck for the two-hour trip. On the drive home, they tell me how they've set up the downstairs so I can get around. Though I'm no longer stuck in a hospital and getting poked with needles, I still have a very long road of recovery looming ahead. I have no idea what the future will be like. I can only focus on the present. I look out the window, watching the soft, cotton-white clouds float by in the bright blue sky. I feel the warmth of the sun on my face slightly magnified through the glass window. I roll down the window so the fresh air can penetrate the deepest spaces in my weakened lungs. The humid summer air is mixed with the car exhaust and diesel fumes from the other vehicles on the road. I inhale deeply, missing the smell of the real world that bypassed me this summer.

Sitting in the front passenger seat and gazing out the window, I know I am returning home. But what exactly am I returning to? I sourly reflect upon two athletic goals I had made at high school graduation. I was all set to swim for St. Mary's College. Now it's doubtful that I'll ever be able to swim again, considering the damage done to my shoulder, pelvis, and lungs. I had also wanted to compete in an Ironman triathlon. But instead of swimming 2.4 miles, biking 112 miles, and running 26.2 miles, my new triathlon will consist of brushing my teeth, combing my hair, and using the toilet by myself.

I lower my eyes to meet the outside side mirror. My face looks thin, pale, and haggard. I don't look eighteen, but more like a tired eighty-eight-year-old man. My cheekbones are practically poking through my skin. I barely have any fat left in my face. My nose looks like skin wrapped tightly over cartilage. Dark circles cradle my bloodshot eyes. I must learn to accept the foreign me.

As we begin driving down our street, my parents warn me that the wrecked Camaro is parked in the driveway near the woods that border our house. It was towed there after the accident. I nervously shoot a glance at the crumpled black hulk as we approach it. Where a driver's seat used to be is gone, pancaked out of existence.

My dad parks and carries me into the house, down the hallway and then toward the living room where he places me carefully on the couch. After bringing in the rest of my stuff from the truck, he goes upstairs to my room and brings down the mattress and bed frame into the living room. This will be my new bedroom. My dad moves the couch to the left side of the bed where my mom is going to sleep, and he aligns the reclining chair to be on the bed's right side. This is where he is going to sleep. Even though I don't have twenty-four-hour nurses anymore, I am sandwiched between two very concerned parents. I feel finally safe, at peace.

I'M AMAZED AT HOW DIFFERENT THE HOUSE LOOKS. ALL THE WALLS HAVE been recently painted but every room seems to be in total chaos—clothes thrown all over the floor, papers scattered across tables. I ask my mom what happened, and she explains that all their focus has been on me. I feel a small surge of guilt but realize how utterly dependent I am on them for everything. I still need their help to make the short walk to the bathroom. I try to use the cane, but my balance is shaky and not to be trusted.

One of my biggest worries is how much weight I have lost. I went from 230 pounds to 130 pounds. Most of that hundred pounds was muscle. Being bulked-up might have saved my life. I heard a doctor once remark that my body had been feeding off all the muscle mass when I was in the coma. Another doctor mentioned that my extra body weight at the accident site gave my internal organs cushion from the several tons of impact that slammed into the left side of my body.

So there are two things that require immediate addressing: gaining back the weight and building up muscles. It's too early for my system to start gulping down protein shakes like I used to do for quick weight gain before track season. So I start with the muscles. With my parents watching television, I begin doing the seven different arm and leg exercises like I did at Kernan.

I slowly go through the first set, experiencing the familiar burning sensation of inactive muscles being worked. I push past the intense pain, but I know I must force myself to be even tougher than when "no pain, no gain" was my mantra as a weightlifter and swimmer. This is a different kind of pain, because my survival and independence depend on it. Unrestricted by the fluorescent, antiseptic confines of the hospital— no more needles, paralysis, seizures, life support, being fed through a tube—I now have to take control of my own destiny. But how is this even possible? How far am I willing to go in order to repair my shattered body?

After my workout is done, the day's excitement has tired me. I try to fall asleep but I can't get comfortable in my bed. I've become so used to stiff, crinkly hospital mattresses, where every move your body makes sounds like you're lying upon a wrestling mat covered in potato chips. I'm disappointed because I've been looking forward to sleeping in my soft bed, but the box springs are pushing into my spine and when I turn over, gravity puts too much weight on my back, which causes problems with my breathing.

I finally discover a comfortable position by lying upon my back with my arms spread out to the sides, which is the position I was forced to adopt in the hospital because I usually had IVs in both arms and a blood pressure cuff. My mattress crucifixion comes home.

I wake up several times throughout the night, tossing and turning, expecting to be accosted at any minute by a nurse ready to jab a needle in my arm to take blood. Then I hear the sound of the lawn mower start up. It's not a dream. I glance at the clock. It's 3:00 a.m. I look over at my mom; she's still asleep. But my dad is gone. He's outside mowing the lawn in pitch darkness. Has he lost his mind?

I'VE BEEN AWAY FROM THE COMPUTER ALL SUMMER. AND NOT BY CHOICE. I'm curious what awaits me in the email inbox. Holding onto the walls for support, I hobble over to the den to my computer. My mom brings me in a pillow because my tailbone remains sensitive.

The moment I sign onto AOL Instant Messenger, I find messages from everybody—friends, relatives, and strangers who have been following my progress on the website that my Uncle Chip and Aunt Lisa put together when I was in the hospital. I'm overwhelmed by their concern and support.

While juggling several simultaneous conversations, I check the email but there are so many unread messages in the inbox that the computer crashes. I reboot the system and locate several hundred emails. As I begin reading the messages, I become emotional and start crying. These emails touch my heart, the same heart that a collision with a dump truck on July 6 rudely shoved across my chest, the heart that stopped beating in Intensive Care, the heart that somehow managed to keep me alive through the infections and coma, the heart that is beating now so that I can sit at my computer and read these wonderful words.

From my high school principal, Garth Bowling, on July 27, 2004:

Dear Mr. and Mrs. Boyle,

I am so sorry to hear about Brian's car accident. He is such a wonderful young man and I know how proud you are of him. We at McDonough High School are all hoping and praying that he will have a full recovery. Many of us have been reading the website so we can keep updated on Brian. I will keep him in my daily thoughts and prayers. Please let us know if we can be of any help.

From my Uncle Joey, Aunt Donna, and younger cousin Garrett on September 1, 2004:

Brian,

We love you! Glad you're feeling better—can't wait until you come home. With your positive attitude all things are possible.

From one of my very good childhood friends, Molly Simpson, on September 4, 2004:

Brian,

I'm so glad to keep hearing how great you are doing! It amazes me to read your progress from day to day. I'm leaving tomorrow for college, but I will keep in touch and come see you when you are ready to have visitors. Keep it up!

From my Aunt Lisa, Uncle Chip, and cousins Ethan, Wyatt, and Sydney on August 26, 2004:

Brian,

Your mom and dad have been updating us on your progress every day and we are so glad to hear how well you are doing. Uncle Chip can't wait to take you to meet Godsmack in October. We are so excited for you to finally go home. We love you and keep you in our prayers everyday.

From one of my good friends, Rachel Gearhart, on August 28, 2004:

Just want you to know that I think you're pretty wonderful! I'm so glad you're feeling better! I love you, sweetie!

From my biggest rival on the high school swim team and good friend, Josh Turner, on September 10, 2004:

Brian,

Man, sorry to hear the bad news. But I read that you're making progress. I expect you to compete against me again some day and you're only going to be better from all of this, so I'll bring my best. I'm going to come see you before I'm off to school and that's a promise, bro. Hang in there, dude. I'll see you soon. All my prayers.

From my high school art teacher, Mrs. Eicholtz, on September 5, 2004:

Brian,

I'm so glad to hear that you're doing so well! All the teachers at McDonough have been praying for you. As you recoup, your love for art will be a nice outlet for you. The skills you learned in high school will help you to create; I really think you are the one student who enjoyed and explored the most in your advanced level art class this year. And, congrats on being the highest scorer on the art portfolio; zoning in on your concentration early in the year was what really made your portfolio so great! As you heal and feel up to it, let me know if I can get you any art supplies or anything. My prayers are with you always.

From my really great friend and fellow swimmer, Sam Fleming, on September 7, 2004:

Brian,

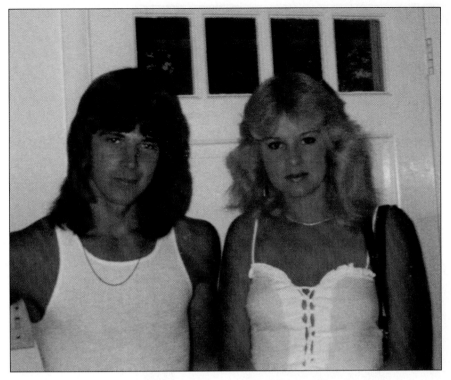

Mom and Dad, in 1977, on their way to a Led Zeppelin concert. My eighteenth year didn't go as well as theirs.

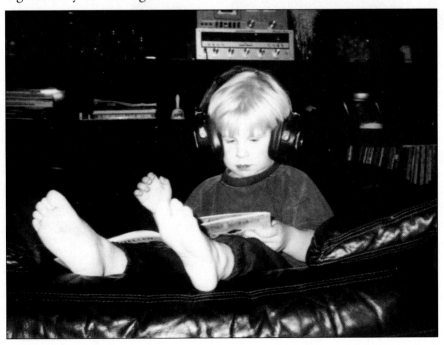

Dad had an extensive record collection of rock classics. Here I am at four years old, listening.

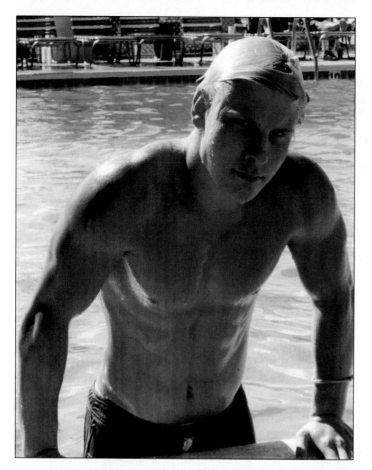

Summer of 2001, my sophomore year, age fifteen, when I began my competitive high school swimming career. One of the best choices I ever made.

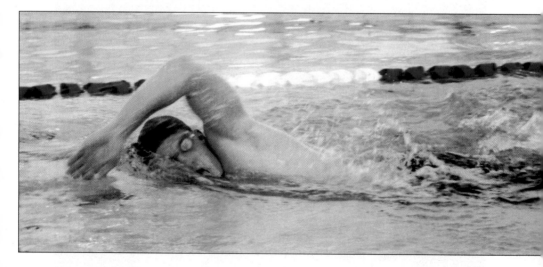

Swimming laps. I really miss my high school swimming days; there were a lot of great memories.

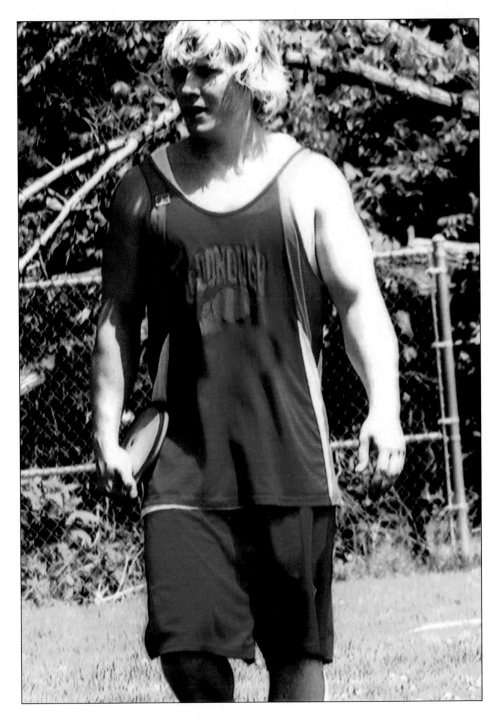

Getting ready to throw the discus in a high school meet in May 2004, which was about a month and a half before the accident. I bulked up to 230 pounds at this point in the season.

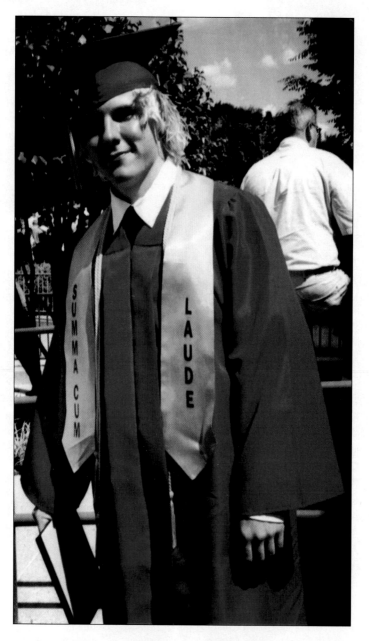

High school graduation day. I was really proud of what I had accomplished both academically and athletically. I was ready for the future, or so I thought.

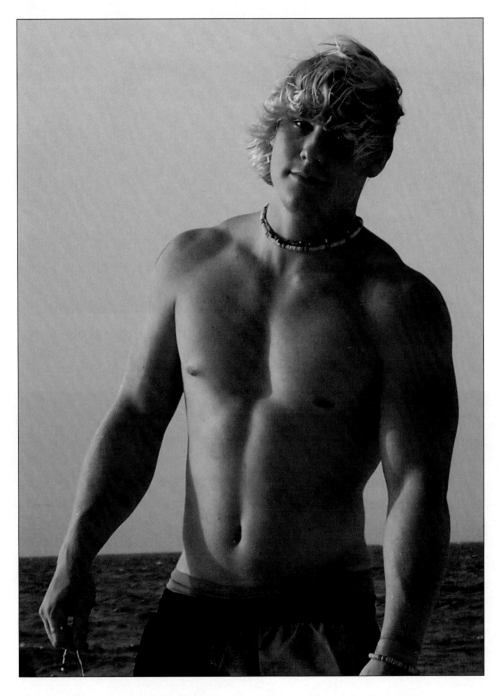

In Jamaica for my senior graduation trip. Two weeks before the accident.

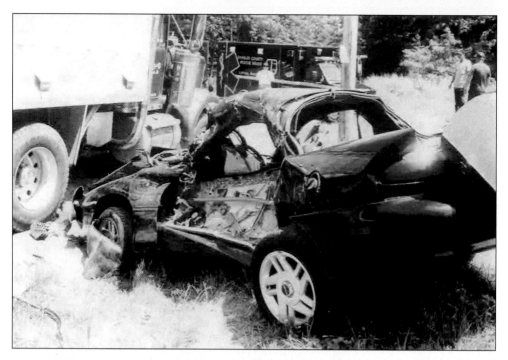

July 6, 2004. My smashed-up Camaro. This crash-scene photo is haunting.

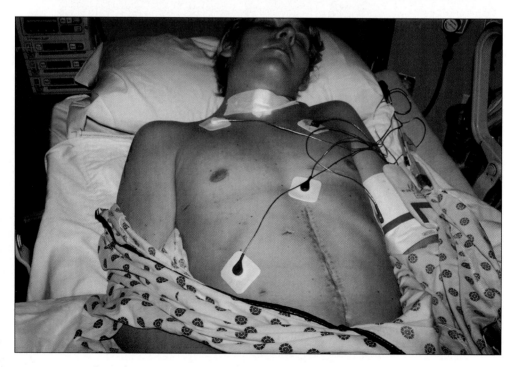

My last day in Intensive Care before being moved up to the eighth floor. The tracheotomy tube had just been removed from my throat.

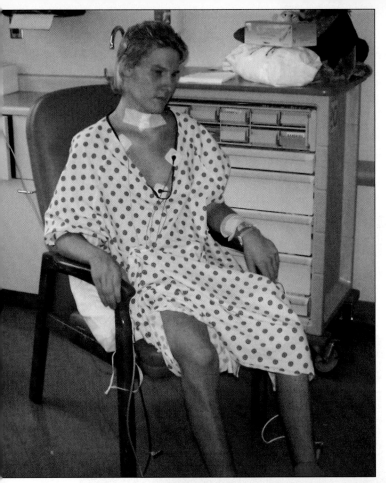

Depressed and discouraged, I had lost one hundred pounds by this point. I feel like a skeleton boy.

My towering medical file. My parents were always signing papers authorizing surgery and treatment.

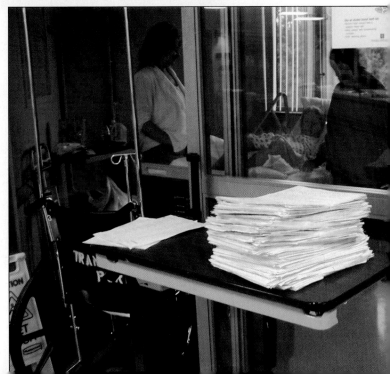

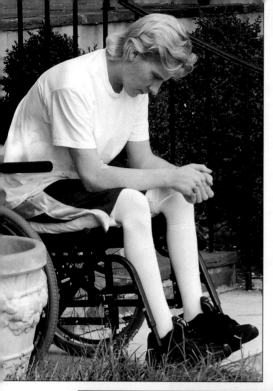

My first day at the rehab center in Baltimore. Looking down at my broken body, I can only think, "Lord, where do I go from here?" Full recovery and a normal life seem impossible.

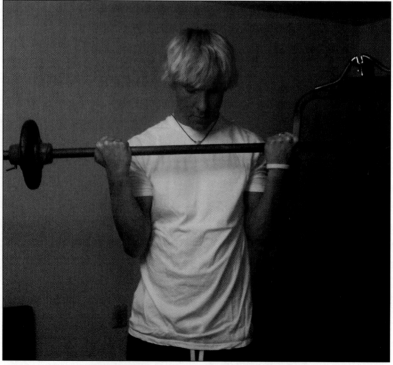

Six months after getting out of the hospital. I used to be able to bicep-curl 50 pounds with each arm for repetitions, and now I struggle to lift the barbell with five-pound plates on each side. This is hard, psychologically and physically.

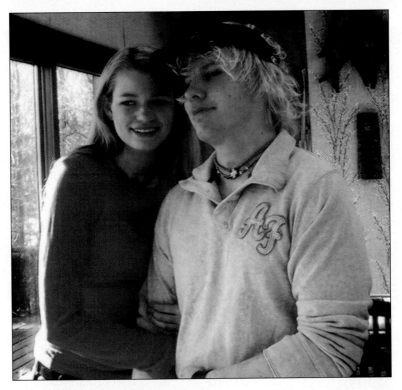

Me and Rachel Gearhart, a special person and friend. She was there for me through both good times and bad.

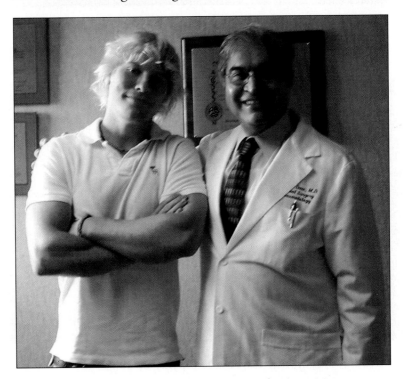

Me and Dr. Daee, my trauma surgeon, July 6, 2005.

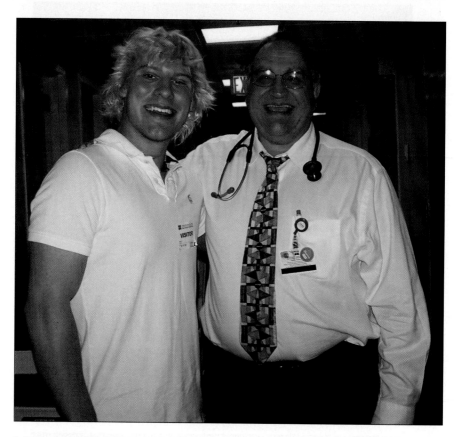

Me and Dr. Catevenis, my Intensive Care doctor, July 6, 2005.

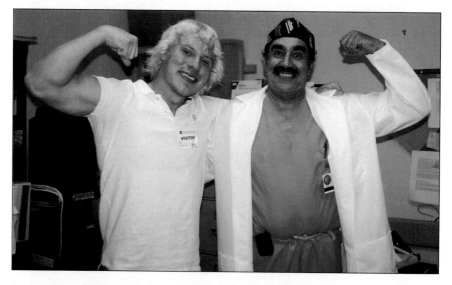

Me and Dr. Naficy, my heart surgeon, July 6, 2005.

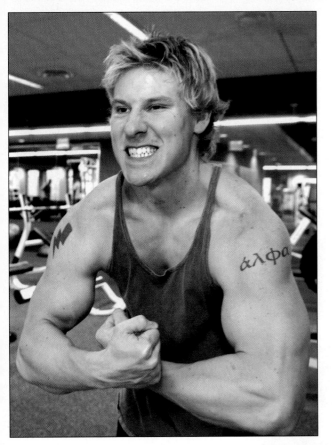

Bulking up at the gym two years after leaving the hospital. The bodybuilding passion is back and bigger than ever.

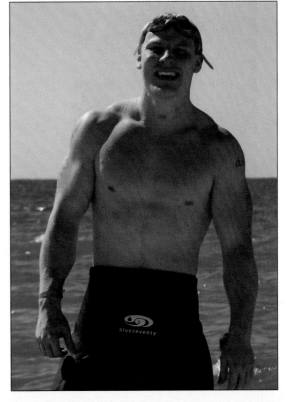

August 2007—From bodybuilding to triathlon. About to go for a practice swim on the day before the Steelhead 70.3 half-Ironman in Lake Michigan. One racer waded by me and said, "With all those muscles, you might sink to the bottom."

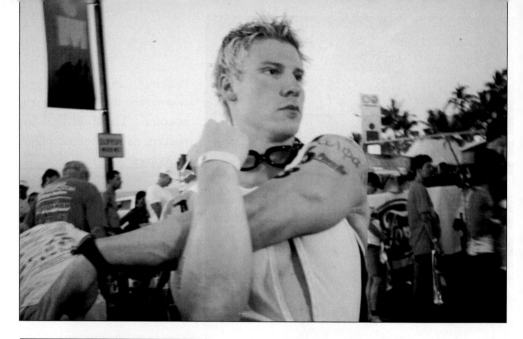

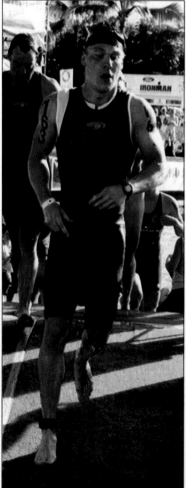

October 2007—Just before the swim start at the Hawaii Ironman in Kona.

I had a good Ironman swim—one hour, 11 minutes for 2.4 miles.

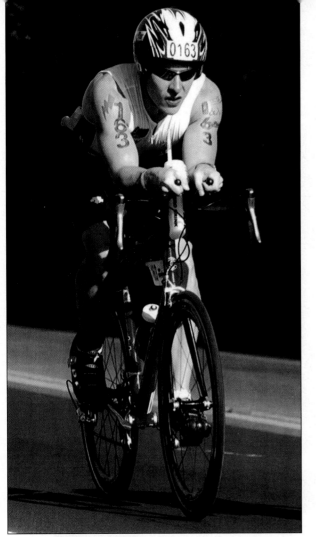

Riding my Cannondale on the Queen K Highway—long, hot, desolate. A ride I will never forget.

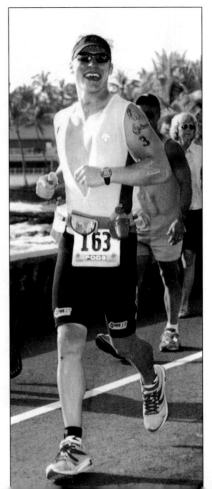

Running through town during the early section of the marathon. That smile on my face doesn't last long once I make it onto the Queen K.

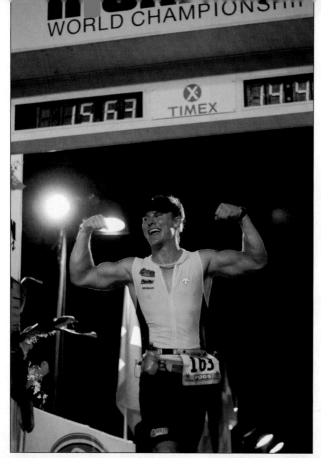

The best day of my life—crossing the Hawaii Ironman finish line.

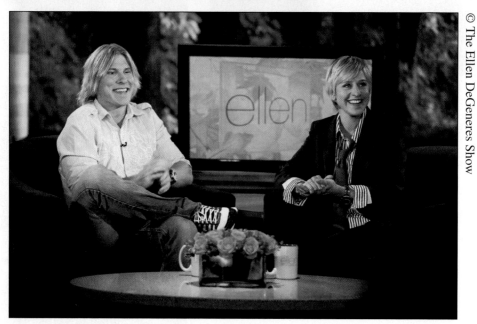

Ellen DeGeneres's talk show lifted my spirits while I was hospitalized. Little did I know that one day I'd be a guest on her show.

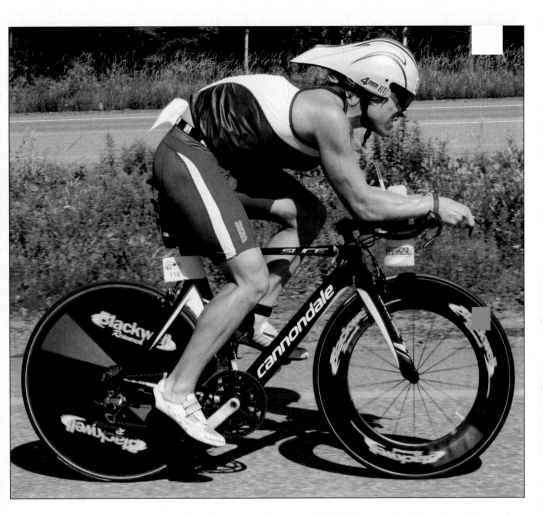

Summer 2008—Riding my new Cannondale Slice at the Newfoundland 70.3 half-Ironman. The tricked-out bike was given to me for receiving the Cannondale Determination Award in 2007.

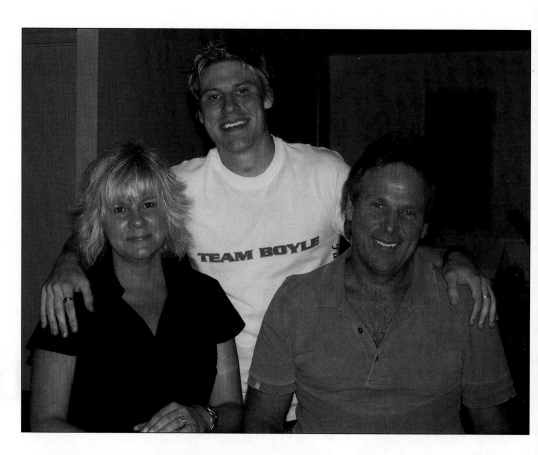

A happy family again, three days after returning home from the Hawaii Ironman in October 2007. Not sure where the journey will take us, but we are grateful for having come this far.

Dude, You are the most inspirational person I've ever met. Keep staying strong, bud! Whenever you're ready to swim just give me a call and I'll be there. And anytime you want to hang or workout, I'll be there. Take care, bud!"

From the Omaha, Nebraska, rock group 311, on August 28, 2004:

Being positive is real easy when things are going great, but it's the real test when the fit hits the shan. Life is a gift, and to be here enjoying it is the meaning of life. We are here and we don't know why; so, learn as much as you can, treat people right, and enjoy this precious gift. We are all family. No one is just a fan to us; we know that everyone is divine. The new album is going to be right up your alley, with contemplative leanings on the dark side, lyrically (dealing with breakups and bad attitudes), and of course a good mixture of hard jams and mellow reggae grooves, with some experimental rock in there for good measure.

From U.S. Olympic Swimmer, Gary Hall Jr., on September 10, 2004:

A hello and welcome back from one swimmer to another. I had a chance to read up on the terrible accident on your family's website. As sorry as I was to hear about your misfortune, I am just as, if not more, relieved to hear that things are returning back to normal and that you, through unimaginable determination, are picking up the pieces. For this I offer my most sincere congratulations. You have my respect and admiration. I was very impressed with your enthusiasm for life. Obviously, it has assisted you back to health. Your grades, your swimming, your writing portray a tremendous human being, one of the good ones. This is perhaps what makes your accident such a tragedy. The world needs people like you. We can't afford to lose you. Particularly moving was the Charles Dickens quote on your website: "Ride on! Rough shod if need be. Smooth shod if that will do, but ride on! Ride on over all obstacles and win the race!" Welcome back. I look forward to one day meeting you; maybe we'll go for a swim. Ride on.

From my cousin and close friend, Matt Mansfield, on September 1, 2004:

Brian Boyle—he walks, he talks, and even uses his muscles again! You showed everyone what Divine Intervention really is, what a miracle is, what happens when you really mean something in this world, and mean something to other people. You showed your family, your doctors, and your friends, that it can happen to anyone. The way I look at it is that you are just starting your life as a smart, strong, healthy, friendly, and the definition of a happy and dedicated person. You are the symbol of living life stronger than death. You are the strongest person I know and probably will ever know. You are my cousin, my best friend, my big brother. I love you bro, and always will.

From my cousin and close friend, Hayley Mansfield, on September 1, 2004:

Brian . . .

I'm so excited you're doing better! And, I can't wait to see you! You are such an incredible and caring person, and this past summer you have taught me so much about life. You taught me that things happen in life that you can't explain. They just happen and have no reason for it. Nobody knew that when they said goodbye, it was almost forever. No one knows how strong you really are, how much you can fight the pain, but you proved you get through anything. This isn't the battle, but it is the war. You have to fight stronger than you ever have before. Each day that goes by gets more intense. The question isn't anymore if you'll make it; it's how much longer it will take. You prove that miracles do happen, that the power of prayer is so much. You prove there is a God out there. You taught me not only to never give up on my dreams, but to never give up on myself. This, I believe, keeps you going every day. This keeps you strong. It shows you the most important things in life. This isn't over; it will never be. But you will stay strong; you will overcome this. I look up to you through all of this. Brian, you are my hero.

I turn off the computer and sit in silent, teary awe. My mom notices that I have been crying. "Everything okay, honey?" she asks.

"Life couldn't be greater," I respond. I really mean this.

DURING MY FIRST FEW DAYS HOME, I RELAX WHEN I'M NOT PUSHING through exercise routines. I watch a lot of daytime television like the *Ellen DeGeneres Show, Andy Griffith Show,* and ESPN's *SportsCenter,* and favorite movies like *Butch Cassidy and the Sundance Kid, Patton, Easy Rider, Stand By Me, Goodfellas,* and *Jeremiah Johnson.* I'm also reading and rereading all the letters and get-well cards that I received from family and friends when I was in the hospital.

Most afternoons, my parents guide me to the back porch for fresh air. I sit back in the cushioned lounge chair and enjoy watching the autumn breeze flow through the leafy branches of the cedar, oak, and dogwood trees in our backyard. When I was little, my dad and I used to go for long walks in the same woods that I'm looking at now.

One day, my good friend Rachel from high school visits. In my frail state, I feel embarrassed. She's extremely attractive. I want to jump off the porch and hide under the bushes. I don't want anybody to see me like this. But her warmth and caring quickly melt away any anxiety. It turns out that she is well past shock—she visited me at the hospital many times, though I have no memory of this.

Rachel begins stopping by the house several times a week. I enjoy her company. She never makes me self-conscious about my appearance. She even begins thinking about becoming a nurse.

Every Tuesday and Thursday, I'm scheduled to attend physical and occupational outpatient therapy sessions at the Child and Adult Rehabilitation Center, which is located about thirty minutes from home. As soon as my parents wheel me into this place, I know that I am going to like it.

The woman at the desk politely gives us a quick tour of the center, which is slightly larger than a regular doctor's office. The focus is on individualized treatment. My first therapist is a pleasant sixty-year-old woman named Carroll. She's tall, nearly six feet, with short dyed-blonde hair, and a constant smile.

We start with improving my balance, since standing unassisted will help me walk on my own. She suggests yoga and tai chi moves. This works well because I practiced yoga while on my high school swim team. Our coach was an Olympic swimmer from Czechoslovakia who wanted me to be more flexible and fluid in the water.

Carroll has me sit on a pillow on a small wooden bench as I try to follow along with the tai chi and yoga routines from a DVD playing on the television. Even as I'm stressing my body, there's a meditative quality that lessens the pain.

I spend my second hour of physical therapy with a black athletic woman named Tosheeda who used to run track in her home country of Jamaica. I love her Caribbean accent. "Hey, mon, I know you can lif' da weight with your leg. Push, mon, push!" She is more aggressive than Carroll. It's like I have a yin and yang team on my side.

Even though the weights that Tosheeda straps to my ankles are only two and a half pounds each, my calves and quads ache after several leg lifts. Then she straps the weights to my arms. Throughout each set of arm raises, she carefully monitors my blood pressure. By the time I finish, I'm drenched in sweat.

On Thursdays, I have occupational therapy with the gentle, calm Cameele, who is pursuing a post-graduate degree and works part-time in the mornings. We do exercises that will help restore the nerves in my left arm and shoulder. These include rolling a rubber ball up a wall and raising and lowering my left arm. She also uses an E-Stem, which is a nerve stimulation device that will help reactivate (I hope) the nonworking nerves in my shoulder that were damaged by the dump truck slamming into the driver's side of the Camaro. The nerves are stimulated by tiny electrical impulses that travel from the equipment box to conductive patches on my arm and shoulder. I feel a slight tingling sensation as the muscle fibers are zapped from the low voltage. Cameele says that when people have severe nerve damage in their shoulder, they usually don't have feeling in their fingers. But somehow I'm able to move my fingers, hand, and forearm.

My first week of outpatient therapy goes much better than expected. Despite the prospect of many months, if not several years, of therapy, working with these three wonderful women won't make it so bad.

My chief concern, however, is with my dad, whose behavior has become odd and erratic. He barely speaks to us. He walks around the house with a blank look, unsmiling and constantly tense. He will stare for hours at the television even when it's not turned on. Often he has difficulty breathing, and I catch him clutching his chest in discomfort.

He won't tell me or my mom what's wrong. He becomes defensive and angry whenever we ask.

He's completely different from the person who would remain in my hospital room, while my mom would run out crying. For some inexplicable reason, their roles have reversed. She's the strong one now. He has emotionally shut down as if he has post-traumatic stress. The strong family warrior has turned into a shell-shocked returning vet—listless, moody, with an invisible injury draining him of vitality.

I begin to think that he's angry with me, that he's having trouble accepting the fact that I'm just a five-eleven big baby who needs constant care. I regularly do my breathing exercises with an inspirometer device, but now I don't want him to watch me struggle to get the little blue ball to rise in the plastic tube. One late morning, I'm working the inspirometer and achieve my personal best for a single breath: a quarter of the way to the gauge's top. My dad is in the kitchen with my mom, but I know he's eyeing me. He then walks over to my bed and wants to know how difficult it is to get the blue ball to rise to the top. I hand him the device so he can find out for himself. He aligns the tube and inhales. The blue ball rises so fast it almost cracks the plastic tube. He gives me back the inspirometer without saying anything. He walks away, his right hand rubbing his chest, but instead of heading to the kitchen, he goes outside so he can be alone on the back porch.

What was that all about? Why is he so troubled? Is there anything I can say to lift his spirits and return him to our family? Does he need to hear the same kind of tough-love speech he gave me in Intensive Care when I was ready to call it quits?

I decide to speak with him, but first I have to get out of bed. I carefully lift my bony legs over the side of the bed, listening to the joints pop, as I rest my feet on the carpet. I have trouble standing up, even as I push off the bed with my arms. I will have to crawl. I go ten feet when I see my dad through the sliding glass door as he sits in a picnic table chair under an umbrella. He's simply staring at the sky. There is such sadness in his eyes. His hand is over his chest and he looks pale. All of a sudden he turns in my direction and our eyes meet. Right then, my mom appears in the living room and sees me on the floor. She screams and tries to help me up, but I quickly tell my mom to go help my dad instead because he looks like he is having a heart attack. She runs outside, then darts back inside to call 911.

Three paramedics arrive within minutes. They rush over to me because I'm still lying on the floor, but I tell them to go outside because my dad is the one in grave danger. They sprint out to the porch with their duffel bags of medical gear. They strap a blood pressure cuff around his arm, while checking his vitals and asking him questions. Two more paramedics race around the rear of the house pushing a gurney toward my dad. As soon as they get to him, they gently lift him onto it and wheel him back through the house. My dad looks down at me on the carpet and says that he loves me. The room begins spinning. It's almost like a tornado has just come down from the sky, snatching up my dad in a flash, then whirling away.

Mom comes running down the stairs and quickly helps me get off the floor and into my shoes. She grabs my hand and guides me to the garage to her white Nissan Xterra SUV. She assists me into the passenger seat, then lugs the heavy wheelchair into the trunk and lays it flat on its side. She speeds out of the driveway, kicking up dirt and gravel as we follow the ambulance that is already several minutes down the road.

We get to the local hospital called Civista Medical Center, which is only fifteen minutes from home. My mom jumps out of the car, taking out the wheelchair from the trunk and placing it on the ground. She comes around on the passenger side where I'm sitting and helps me out. I can't keep up with her frantic actions, so she slows down and gets me situated in the wheelchair. She pushes me across the parking lot and up onto the sidewalk and into the emergency area. We head straight to the front desk to see where my dad is. The young female receptionist says that they are currently running several tests on him and that we should take a seat.

My mom wheels me over to the corner of the room and positions me next to two open seats by a set of red double doors that lead into the inner dwellings of the emergency unit. I lower my head in my hands in disbelief. When are we ever going to get a break? I peek between my fingers to see who else is in the waiting room. A young boy is resting an ice pack on his knee, a middle-aged woman is holding a baby in her arms, and an older man has white gauze covering part of his head. All this waiting, even if it's only minutes, fills me with anxiety about my dad's health. And to think: this is what my parents did for months—wait and wait and wait.

A half hour passes and still no news. My mom browses a celebrity gossip magazine but I can tell she's agitated. A woman comes walking through the double doors and stops right in front of us. She's wearing a blue EMT uniform. She has short grayish-blonde hair, glasses, and is smiling. She seems to know me, but I have no idea who she is.

"You must be Brian Boyle. I'd recognize that beach blond hair anywhere," she says. "My name is Dawn-Moree Dugan and I'm the Assistant Chief for the Ironsides Volunteer Rescue Squad. I was at your accident scene. Boy, you were a fighter. You were the second strongest person our crew ever dealt with, the first being a 250-pound Maryland sheriff. So give me a hug, handsome!"

I slowly get up and give Dawn a well-deserved hug, while profusely thanking her for saving my life even though I have no memory of what happened. I ask her what she remembers.

"Well, Brian, a majority of the people who are hit the way you were die in their vehicle right then and there at the accident scene. They may have been struck by a small car or SUV and do not make it. But you were hit by a dump truck and survived! It's almost unbelievable. You were trapped in your seat and even the Jaws of Life couldn't extricate you. We had to remove your shorts and swimsuit for your body to slide out. You had to be rushed to Prince George's Hospital trauma unit within minutes. The medevac guys thought that was all the time that you had left because of the massive blood loss."

Dawn pauses and stares intensely at me. "I'm looking at you right now and I'm absolutely amazed. I can't believe it. There were so many things that could have gone wrong that day, but you made it through. It is safe to say that luck was definitely on your side."

Dawn can't stay because she has to leave on a 911 call. Someone just fell off a ladder at his house. She gives me another hug and tells me to stop by the Rescue Squad when my dad feels better.

Her words leave me wondering: How or why did I survive the crash? Think of all the odds stacked up against me. The Camaro could have caught on fire with me still in it. The gas tank was on the driver's side, and that was where the dump truck slammed into me. What if I hadn't been wearing a seat belt? Which window would I have flown through from the impact? But the seat belt saved my life, despite breaking my clavicle. What if the rescue team hadn't been able to get me out of the car in time? What if there hadn't been a helicopter to take me to Prince George's Hospital? The local hospital where I'm at now could not have saved me because they don't have the technology.

Finally, the girl at the front desk signals to us that we can see my dad. My mom pushes me in the wheelchair through the red double doors as we follow a nurse down a long empty hallway until we reach a small room with a pink cloth divider. An old man is sleeping in one bed, with an oxygen tube under his nose. I look past him and see my dad's shoes poking out from the other side of the pink divider. We go around the curtain, and there he is—lying in the bed with his shirt off and several electrodes attached to various areas of his chest, arms, and lower neck. He appears calm, but his bloodshot eyes tell another story. He says that the doctors ran several tests on his heart and did some blood work, and they ruled out a heart attack. It turned out to be a panic attack caused by stress and anxiety.

Mom sits down in the chair next to him. I remain in my wheelchair, wishing I could do something to make him feel better and reduce his stress. What did he always do when I was in Room 19 to make me feel better? I know. I untie his shoes and slide them off his feet. He shoots me a curious look because he's unsure what I'm doing. I start rubbing his feet, and we both begin laughing.

CHAPTER 20

THE TRACK

My parents encourage me to leave the house with them when they go out for errands. But the day trips to Home Depot and Lowe's fail to excite me because I have to be pushed around in a wheelchair. Shopping makes me self-conscious. I feel strangers' eyes bore right through me and see all the scars zigzagging across my neck, chest, and stomach. I definitely look sickly. My hair is falling out. The doctors told me that this might happen because of all the medication that had flooded my system. Home and the therapy center are the only two places where I don't feel like a freak.

On the bright side, I'm gaining weight. The doctors monitor my protein intake on a weekly basis to make sure that my body is able to process it. There's a real concern because my gall bladder and spleen were removed. They give me the green light to consume whey protein powders like I used to take when transforming from swimmer to discus thrower. There are several jugs of protein already in our kitchen closet, and I quickly go through them. My parents take me to one of the vitamin stores, where we spend a small fortune on multiple containers, but I know the money is well spent. More weight and muscle equals more strength.

I now drink two protein shakes with my meals. Along with the shakes, I also eat two protein bars. I'm getting about 150 grams of protein a day. The interesting thing about consuming all that protein is that you have to exercise to turn it into muscle—otherwise it will be stored as excess fat. I learned this lesson in my sophomore year when I tried to put on weight too quickly, thinking that the protein powder would magically turn into muscle all by itself. That's what the magazine ads always said. But I became bloated instead.

MY YOUNGER COUSINS MATT AND HAYLEY, WHO LIVE IN ANNAPOLIS, like coming over to hang out. Matt just started high school and Hayley is still in middle school, and they are the brother and sister I never had and always wanted. Matt and I are similar in many respects. We act the same, talk the same, and very much look the same—but with different color hair. We grew up together, played the same sports, and listened to the same music. We could read each other's thoughts, and we both prefer to keep our feelings to ourselves.

Every day when my parents would leave the hospital, my mom would always update my Aunt Kati, her sister, about my condition. Kati would then relay the information to my Uncle Tom and then to Hayley and Matt, but Matt would never want to hear the news. He refused to accept that his cousin and best friend was dying. The first time he came to see me in the hospital, he brought me his personal CD player with some Jimi Hendrix CDs. I was the one responsible for introducing him to Jimi and he thought that I would be able to listen to him. But at that time, I was deathly ill and still in a coma.

Hayley later told me that while I was in the hospital, her brother would sit in his bedroom all day and work on art that was dedicated to me. His art included digital photography of swimming idols, rock legends, mythological beings like Thor, and comic-book icons like Iron Man. Hayley would write down thoughts in her journal. If the news about my condition was good that day, she would jump up and down with happiness. If it was bad, there would be tears of sadness.

Now that I'm home and spending a lot of time with Matt and Hayley, I can tell that the accident has taken a psychological toll on her because she is so young. She began having panic attacks whenever she went outdoors because in the back of her mind she constantly thought that what happened to me could also happen to her. I tell her that we don't have the power to decide what will happen to us today or tomorrow, but we do have the power to decide how we can react to those events.

On weekends when they visit, we watch movies together. They help me do my exercises, listen to me when I need someone to talk to, and every time I have to get up to walk somewhere they are on both sides of me, making sure I get there safely.

My grandmother and grandfather on my mom's side, whom I call Nana and Big D, have also been a great help and brighten my mood. I think the reason that I love art is because Nana inspired me to be creative and use my imagination at an early age. She loved telling me stories about what it was like growing up in Newfoundland. But with her diabetes and other ailments growing worse, we now mostly talk about medical matters.

Joe Lineberger, my grandfather, is called Big D, which is short for Big Daddy. He was born in Maiden, North Carolina, in 1931. His first job was picking cotton in the fields, and the few cents he earned each week he gave to his mother. He excelled in academics and athletics and was accepted by Duke University, where he had to work two jobs to pay for his schooling. In 1953, he entered the Air Force as a second lieutenant through the Reserve Officer Training Corps program. He served in overseas assignments that included Thule Air Base in Greenland, Pepperell Air Force Base in Newfoundland, exchange duty with the Royal Canadian Air Force in Ottawa, and Headquarters Military Assistance Command in South Vietnam.

He accomplished all of this with a wife and five children and is now one of the highest-ranked officers at Andrews Air Force Base. I use his successful background and career as motivation to fortify my own determination to resume a regular life.

The first step back to normalcy is liberation from the wheelchair. I have gone from standing for several minutes to hobbling the fifteen feet from my bed to the kitchen table. I stop and rest, then shuffle back to the bed. Several hours later, I do it again. Soon, I'm able to walk further. One regular trip is the twenty-five feet from the hallway door to the garage. I'd get to the doorknob, stop and rest, and then return to my bed. The most difficult part about learning how to walk again is stairs. Once my foot makes it onto the first step, I have to catch my breath, rest, and five minutes later I do the same with my left foot. Descending steps is just as tiring and laborious.

For two consecutive months, I focus my energy and attention on walking. It means freedom from my two-wheel fortress of dependent mobility. Even though I have to stop to take a break every few minutes,

I find immense joy and pleasure in walking on my own two feet. With constant exercises, stretches, plyometrics, and an incredible amount of balance drills, I'm finally able to permanently graduate from the wheelchair to a cane. It's a relief not having to ask my mom or dad for a sandwich or to grab a clean T-shirt from my room.

Within several weeks, I no longer need a cane to move around. As my legs get stronger, there comes additional motivation to speed up rehab, as if a chain reaction has been set into motion. I decide to immerse myself in the atmosphere of a real gym. When I was on my high school swim team, I did a lot of cardio work. I would ride the stationary bike, run on the treadmill, and do hundreds of ab crunches. In order to get more muscular for discus throwing, I would do bench press sets, pushups, dumbbell workouts, and a lot of powerlifting to build mass. I'd spend hours pumping iron.

My Uncle Joe helps me out at the gym. He works for the Verizon telephone networking system and travels around the area surveying various telephone poles and other communication systems that need his evaluation and approval. During his lunch breaks, he goes to a nearby gym called the Sport & Health Club. So on Tuesdays after therapy, my mom drops me off at the club, which is located only two minutes away from the rehab center. We work out together for about an hour and a half, even though I struggle to lift the lightest weights. My first set of bench presses is with a 25-pound barbell—225 pounds less than I was lifting in June right before the accident. Still, it feels good to be back in a gym, to hear the clanging of iron on iron, the grunts of fellow lifters, the thud when a heavy weight hits the floor.

Now, because of the success of outpatient therapy, there has been a lot of recovery in the nerves in my left shoulder from Cameele's E-stem device. Tosheeda is a miracle worker, helping me regain leg strength. She has me do many of the same drills and regimens that I did on the track team: stretching, high-knee exercises, and simple plyometrics.

One late afternoon, my dad takes me to the high school track for some additional walking. The exercise also benefits him. Ever since his panic attack, he's been taking the antidepressant Zoloft, which has improved his mood. Our first and only lap takes forever, but the track's rubber surface cushions my fragile knees and ankles.

Each week we return to the track. I usually add another lap each time. My dad walks alongside me, which works out well because it gives us more time to talk. We walk at an extremely slow pace. But that's okay. The greatest part is that I am upright, mobile, and not confined to a bed, chair, or cane. Distances are now measured in hundreds of yards rather than several-dozen feet. We seldom discuss the accident. Instead, we focus on my future, since I'm not going to college. I've decided that once my physical therapy is over, I want to learn more about the concrete business. I already know how to operate a concrete pump truck. I'd be following in the footsteps of the family construction business. My dad was always proud of my academic achievements, so it was his dream for me to go to college because he never had the opportunity. But now, I'd rather be around my dad on his different job sites because it'd be therapeutic for him as well.

On our fifth visit to the track, I hear the distant boom of thunder as rain begins falling around us like heavy teardrops. Curiosity consumes me with a burning desire to walk faster. My dad asks me if everything is okay. I nod yes and continue to press on, quickening my pace, almost to the point of losing balance. The faster leg rotations are accompanied by an unexpected lift off from my forefeet as they hit the ground. My walking turns into a slow jog.

I visualize the scene in *Forrest Gump* when he is running away from the bullies as his leg braces fall away. I'm fleeing from the tragedy of July 6 that stole my life. With my unnatural, awkward running style—the slow-to-mend pelvis still causes pain—I must look like an uncoordinated fool. But who cares! I am running! Rain begins splashing upward from the track. My deep gasps play a duet with the sound of each foot striking the wet surface. Walking was once impossible, and now I run.

I jog for another lap before exhaustion finally sets in. I rest my weary body against a fence. Sweat mixes with rain on my face. My dad walks over to me and proudly puts his arms around my shoulder. We both laugh. It's laughter that neither of us wants to cease. I tell him that two laps are good for a start, but what about some day running a mile? My dad starts giggling with happiness. "Brian, don't get too ahead of yourself." It's great to hear the merriment in his voice again.

CHAPTER 21

THE INTERSECTION

DRIVING BACK FROM THE TRACK ONE AFTERNOON, I ASK MY DAD FOR A favor. I want to see the intersection where the accident took place. This will be my first time back there since July 6. He hesitates, but then agrees to the inevitable. He knows I need this closure even though I don't have any recollection of that day.

We take a right onto Ripley Road and follow the winding, two-lane country road for about a mile. The sharp bends come up pretty quickly. We pass over a series of freshly painted rumble strips letting drivers know that a stop sign is ahead at the intersection of Ripley and Poorhouse. We drive a bit further and I see the intersection sign followed by a stop sign. We have arrived at my private Ground Zero. My hands begin to shake. We are both quiet. One would think by our silence that we are paying our respects to the deceased in a cemetery.

My dad parks his truck by the intersection near the grassy embankment that the driver on Ripley sees when he looks to the left, which is the same view I had in the Camaro. The view to the right is worse. The embankments are so overgrown with foliage that you can't see anything until you pull out a few feet beyond the stop sign which then places you directly in the path of oncoming traffic.

We get out of the truck and walk around the accident scene together. I break the silence by asking my dad if he ever spoke to the other driver.

"We never heard from him," he says in anger. "I talked to the investigating officer several times the first week of the accident and all he said was that you were 'smoking tires' and that he was still looking into what happened. I never heard from him after that and none of my phone calls were ever returned."

"Smoking tires? I don't even know how to do that."

My dad responds, "That's because your car is not even able to do that unless you power-brake it."

"Power-brake? What the hell is that?"

My dad looks at me. "Exactly."

"Why would the police even suggest something so false?"

My father thinks they wanted to place the blame on me. But neither of us can guess why.

I ask my dad if he knows anything about the driver. He knows nothing, not even his name. "Cops wouldn't tell us," he says.

My father's rage is palpable. Yet I don't feel any anger toward this mystery driver who wrecked my life and Camaro. How can I? I don't remember the crash. In a way, this phantom driver doesn't even exist. But my scars and damaged body do. The sadness of my parents watching me suffer in the hospital exists. They have been traumatized by the entire ordeal. The local law authorities made it even worse for them by stonewalling and then making up facts.

We watch a green Mustang pull up to the stop sign, coming from the same direction that I was driving from on the day of the accident.

The driver has to nose forward several feet to see if any vehicles are approaching from the left. The front bumper is practically in the middle of the intersection. He finally determines that the road is clear and continues driving on Ripley.

Dad says, "See what I mean about this intersection? It's a safety hazard that the county should have fixed long ago." He tells me that my grandfather and Aunt Kati and Uncle Tom tried to find out what really happened that day. Kati called the investigating officer in July. Apparently, the phone call didn't go well, because as soon as she began asking questions, he became very angry, saying that it was all my fault and that I could have killed someone. He wanted to issue me a fine for failing to remain stopped at the stop sign. He told my aunt that he didn't know if it was a suicide attempt.

I can't believe this nonsense. Suicidal? Me?

"It gets worse," my dad says. "The officer then said that the truck driver mentioned you were playing a game of chicken with him. This was bogus. Aunt Kati also asked him about the police report that said that you were not trapped in the car and that you climbed out of the car all by yourself. And can you believe that the officer said the dump truck driver had to hold you down on the ground because you were combative and flailing about? The investigating officer told your aunt that the truck driver saved your life, which was a lie. She then spoke to another policeman who wasn't involved in the case; fortunately, he was supportive. He said that he couldn't believe that they hadn't put a stoplight at that intersection because it's known to be a dangerous, accident-prone intersection. Something just wasn't right."

Along the side of the road and strewn in the weeds, I look down and see tiny fragments of glass, black paint shards from the Camaro, and a surgical glove with dark bloodstains. Could that be my blood? I bend over and pick up a four-inch piece of a broken outside mirror. I feel its sharp jagged edges. I assume it came from the Camaro.

I walk over to the telephone pole and sit down on a small hill that overlooks the intersection. I stare out at Poorhouse Road, still holding the glass shard. I consider all the what-ifs from that day. If I had swum one additional lap and left the pool one minute later, would the accident still have happened? Or, if the truck driver had an extra cup of coffee at lunch, would we still have met in the middle of Ripley and Poorhouse?

I feel a sharp pinch on my right index finger. I've cut myself on the glass. A small drop of blood has smeared the mirror. The incision is no bigger than a nasty paper cut. I look at the blood, my blood, reconsidering my own mortality. I had almost bled out that day.

I tell my dad that I'm ready to go home.

CHAPTER 22

RETURN TO PRINCE GEORGE'S HOSPITAL

My parents take me over to my Uncle Chip and Aunt Lisa's house in Springfield, Virginia. He's my mom's brother-in-law and works in music management. They want to celebrate my recovery. When I was in the hospital, they created a website so friends and family could check my status.

After dinner, Chip surprises me with the entire collection of the 2004 Athens Olympic Games on VHS. I didn't get to watch much of the Olympics in the hospital, and I only remembered bits and pieces viewed through the thick fog of medication.

My hero from the Games is Gary Hall Jr., who swims the fifty-meter freestyle. I already knew that he won gold, but I have to see the race again. I might never swim again due to my damaged heart, weak lungs, severe nerve damage to my left shoulder, shattered pelvis, and fluid buildup in my lungs, but I'm still inspired by him, especially after that email he sent me.

The fifty-meter freestyle is nothing but pure strength, speed, and adrenaline—and that's why I liked the short distance so much, though in high school it was fifty yards. You need complete confidence and to have your body and mind in total sync before stepping onto the blocks. That combination will get you to the wall before your competitors. Gary is proof of this winning attitude. At age twenty-nine, he touched first in 21.93, beating his Olympic competitors by an eyelash.

I rewind the tape and notice that I missed Gary's prerace interview, which shows clips of him racing at the 2000 Sydney Olympics. He says, "The world's fastest swimmers are in the fifty-meter freestyle. If you are talking about pure speed, I can swim faster than anybody in the world. I've defied doubters time and time again. At first they said I was lazy, undisciplined. This time they're saying, 'Oh you're too old; you can't do it.' I won't go away that easy, so tell me I can't do it. I dare you."

I press the pause button and think about what Gary has just said. If he defied the doubters who believed he could not win, then what's stopping me from getting back in the pool? Not to race, but just to swim again.

Gary's words replay in my mind. That's it, I decide, I'm getting back in the pool. I'm not going to let my injuries limit me. Like Gary, I want to defy the odds.

The next day during my physical therapy, I confide my plan to Carroll, who is thrilled. She says that the best way to get back in the pool would be to transition my yoga and tai chi into the more aquatic version called ai chi, which could be done at an indoor pool. She tells me that when I come back on Thursday for my occupational therapy, she will bring her ai chi VHS tape for me to borrow.

On the drive home from therapy, I explain to my mom why I want to return to swimming. She seems surprised and worried at the same time because of what the doctors had told her. She says that when we get home, she'll schedule an appointment with my doctors to see if we can get their permission.

After we eat lunch, I take a short nap. When I wake, my mom provides unexpected good news. She says that when I was asleep, Andre Barbins, the swim coach from St. Mary's College of Maryland, called asking to see how I was doing because he and the team had been following my progress since the accident. I can't believe the coincidence. He wants to visit and bring the captain of the men's swim team, Julio Zarate. I ask my mom how soon. She looks at me and smiles, "How about tomorrow?"

That night it's hard to sleep. I'm not sure what's wrong; maybe I'm nervous about seeing the coach. My pulse is higher than normal and my breathing is different, labored, like there's a small dog lying on my chest.

Halfway through the night, I have to sit up in my bed to get a full breath of air. I hope it's just a case of anxiety and not something more serious.

The next day, I wake up feeling drowsy and restless from lack of sleep. There's still the pressure on my chest when I breathe and my pulse is racing. In any case, I get ready for Coach Barbins and Julio by putting on my St. Mary's swim team T-shirt.

The first time I met them was in the spring of my senior year about two months before graduation. I was looking at swimming programs at several colleges. When my parents met with Coach Barbins, we felt a genuine connection with him. The school was also only a one-hour drive from home. I soon signed my acceptance papers and would start my freshman year in the fall as one of his top recruits. The accident snuffed out that dream. More than likely, simply being able to float on my back in the pool will be the full extent of my new swimming career.

After lunch, I hear the doorbell ring. It's Coach Barbins and Julio. I struggle to walk to the door, trying to mask my labored breathing because I know my mom can easily detect the slightest problem or ailment and she would insist on taking me to the doctor right away.

We're happy to see Coach Barbins and Julio who present me with T-shirts, a personal letter that the entire team signed, swim caps, training suits, and goggles.

We sit down in the living room and talk about my recovery and my future plans. I mention I'd like to start working with my dad in concrete construction after my physical therapy is over and how I plan to get my Commercial Driver's License in the spring. Right before they leave, Coach Barbins tells me that even though I wasn't able to go to college this semester and swim, I'm still on the team. I hold back tears when I hear this kind offer.

I walk out on the back porch, quietly gasping for breath, and sit down. Mom joins me. "Do you really think I could swim one day?" I ask.

"Honestly, I know you can," she replies without hesitating.

"Yeah, but I mean at a collegiate level?" I say hesitantly, realizing the question's weight.

"Absolutely. I believe that not only will you get back in the pool again, but you'll be great. Look how far you have come already."

"Okay then, let's set up an appointment to get approval from the doctors."

My breathing gets worse at bedtime. I have to sit up the entire night just to capture a small breath of air each time. It feels like I'm drowning and that at any minute I will lose consciousness, have a stroke, or suffer a heart attack. Why are my heart and lungs failing?

In the morning, as I struggle to eat a bowl of cereal at breakfast, I tell my parents about my breathing difficulties. As expected, my mom immediately calls 911.

While I wait for the ambulance to arrive, I shuffle into the bathroom. My balance and equilibrium have deteriorated to the point where I have to hold onto the walls as I move through my house. My vision is distorted and crowded with flickering sparks of light. I close the door behind me and study myself in the mirror. This is it. I've come this far, and now I sense that death has finally caught up to me; it had been slyly waiting in ambush the entire time. It was foolish to think that I could cheat this relentless adversary. Tears begin streaming down my hollow cheeks as Intensive Care memories resurface. Once again, I'm in bed looking up at the all-too-familiar sight of my saddened parents. That image morphs to something bleaker: they are dressed in black and standing over my grave. The tears stream faster. I rest my head in my hands, wishing that things would be different. I don't want to die.

I hear the ambulance's siren, so I hurry to dry my tears and limp back to the living room where I sit on the couch and wait for the two young EMTs to cart me away. But first they check my vital signs. My blood pressure and pulse are extremely high. I'm given an oxygen mask and hooked up to a blood pressure machine. They then lift me onto a gurney and wheel me out the door and into the back of the ambulance. My mom sits in the passenger seat up front, while my dad drives behind us in his truck.

At the Civista Medical Center, I'm rushed into a small room where a nurse begins taking blood samples. She hooks me up to an IV. Five minutes later, a doctor comes in and kindly introduces himself. He requests that I get a CAT scan and chest X-ray. My parents tell him that I suffered severe trauma to my body organs in a motor-vehicle accident over the summer.

I go through all the tests; then we wait. About two hours later, the doctor returns. He's holding a clipboard with papers. He appears confused. Two other doctors also enter the room, both with similarly puzzled expressions. The first doctor says, "Um, Mr. Boyle, we've been looking over your recent scans and we were just wondering what exactly happened to you? Most of your internal organs are not in their correct locations and frankly we have just never seen something like this before. You have nodules and scar tissue all over your lungs, and your heart looks like it has recently undergone a lot of hard work."

My parents explain what happened in greater detail, and everyone comes to the same conclusion that it makes better sense for me to be transferred to Prince George's Hospital where all my medical records are still being held.

My parents help me to the truck and we drive to the hospital. The last time I made the trip here was aboard a helicopter, barely clinging to life.

My parents register me in the regular emergency room. This is a first for all of us, since the medevac helicopter had landed on the hospital roof and I was whisked away to the trauma unit. Judging by the crowded room, it looks like it will be a long wait. A young guy who arrives right behind me is a gunshot victim. He's bent over while holding a dark-with-blood towel over his mouth, with a half-filled bucket at his feet. A buddy is supporting him because he seems as if he's about to pass out.

We wait and wait. All the seats are filled. The air grows stale. It begins to affect my breathing, which is getting more raspy and labored. My heart speeds up. I'm soon gasping for air and motion to my mom that I need help. She jumps up and races over to the front desk. Seconds later, a nurse escorts us to a curtained space within one of the general examination rooms. After I get my blood drawn, I'm injected with an antibiotic solution that slows down my heart and eases my breathing somewhat.

As we wait for a doctor, another nurse comes by to check my vital signs. She says that she remembers me from the summer. She also mentions that a number of staff working in the emergency room tonight might also recall when I was last here at the hospital. She wasn't kidding. Every few minutes, a nurse or hospital employee stops by to introduce him- or herself to me. Some turn emotional talking to us. What's always left unsaid but hangs in the room like a powerful unseen force is that they thought I should be dead.

My parents remember most of their names. I'm amazed by how many people were involved in keeping me alive. I thank them all. It doesn't matter what department they work in or whether they are a top doctor or someone who works part-time in the gift shop; they all played a role in saving me from oblivion.

With all these unexpected well-wishers, I begin to feel dizzy; the only thing that I've eaten all day is a bowl of cereal for breakfast. It's early evening and my stomach has been making annoying noises for the past hour. I ask one of the nurses if I can have something to eat and she walks around the hall and returns with two hospital trays full of food. I thank her and start scarfing down the food. It may be bland hospital grub but it's filling me up.

Bloated yet content, I feel more relaxed. My parents duck out for coffee when the doctor arrives. It's Dr. Daee, the surgeon who first opened me up in the trauma unit. He is chiefly responsible for my continued existence in this world. Within minutes of arriving in the medevac, he made an incision in my chest to see what was wrong and where to start. There was no time to take preliminary X-rays or CAT scans.

Dr. Daee says that he just came from surgery and that he will set me up in the cardiology department to make sure that whatever illness I have will be taken care of quickly, efficiently, and effectively. He adds that he's not surprised to see me back in the hospital because my immune system had been severely weakened from being on life support for so long.

When my parents return and see Dr. Daee, they both give him a big hug. He reassures them that whatever is wrong with me, it's not life threatening. Relief washes over all of us.

Dr. Daee has to meet with the family of the young man he just operated on, so we say our goodbyes.

It takes another half hour for my room to be made up in the cardiology department. A nurse introduces himself to us, pushing a wheelchair that he wants me to sit in. I politely decline his offer, because I can walk on my own, though in reality, I probably should sit down. But it's been my burning desire since the day I left Intensive Care to come back here one day and say hello to everyone while walking on my own. So I take baby steps, huffing and puffing with each short stride, bracketed by the nurse and my parents. He directs us to my room where we are told that only one of my parents can stay overnight with me. After I say goodbye to my dad, the nurse comes back in the room and wraps a heart monitor around my neck and then reconnects my IV to a bag of antibiotics as I lie down on the bed. Another nurse brings in an extra blanket, sheet, and pillow for my mom who will sleep in the recliner chair near the window.

I'm concerned about Mom's emotional state. Did she know that we'd be back in the hospital so soon? What if I really take a turn for the worse? How will she hold up? I'm more frightened for her sake than for my own.

CHAPTER 23

GETTING BACK IN THE POOL

THERE'S NOT MUCH TO DO WHILE I'M BEING CHECKED OVER IN THE cardiology department. Patients are not allowed to leave the floor because our heart rates are constantly monitored. So I've been doing a lot of reading, including biographies of Steve Prefontaine and Lance Armstrong.

Steve, also known as Pre, was America's first running superstar, a James Dean rebel in Nikes, with trademark long hair and mustache. When someone once told him that another runner might beat him in a race, he replied that they would first have to bleed. He died tragically at age twenty-four in a car crash. Pre grew up in Coos Bay, Oregon, near where the fatal wreck occurred. The small marina near my house is called Goose Bay. Just a small rhyming coincidence, but it makes me wonder why he died and I lived.

The word must have spread throughout the hospital that I'm back because familiar and unfamiliar faces begin showing up in my room. "Brian, is that you?" many ask in disbelief. Visitors include nurses, physician's assistants, cleaning ladies, physical and respiratory therapists, and several ICU doctors. It feels like a happy family reunion.

Each one played a part in bringing me back to life, so I go out of my way to tell them how much my parents and I appreciate everything that they did for me. The only thing that I feel bad about is that I wanted everyone to see me walking again, rather than seeing me bedridden.

Dr. Daee looks in on me several times. Dr. Nafisy also stops by. He is the doctor who moved my still-beating heart across my chest when I first arrived in shock trauma. A special aura surrounds him, as if his touch alone heals patients of their illnesses and injuries. Nurses call him "the man with the golden hands."

On the fifth day, Dr. Daee informs me that my breathing problems and elevated heart rate are due to a bacterial infection that caused fluid to build up around my heart and in my lungs. He writes out several prescriptions.

As we wait for my dad to pick us up, there's something I must do. I visit the ICU floor. There are many people who want to say hello. I'm surprised by all the attention I receive—many of the staff have to wait to greet me. Tears moisten many of their eyes.

I ask to see my old room—Room 19. I'm told it's empty, which comes as a relief since I would have hated to see someone suffering there, like I did for over ten weeks. I walk tentatively to the room, and slide open the glass door. The room is all too familiar—same bed, clock on the wall above the door, television in the upper right corner, aqua-cushioned chair, sink that was off-limits to my parched throat, and the high-tech throne of now-silent medical equipment. The window blinds are open and sunshine floods into the room. I approach the sunlit bed. This is where I should have died. I place my left hand on the clean white pillow that awaits the head of the next patient.

Outside the room, my mom is talking to Dr. Catevenis and Dr. Boyce, the ICU directors. I walk out and greet them. They say that I am the most critical patient they've seen who has survived. Both are serious men. I never saw either one smile until my health started to improve. Then, every time they passed my room, these two doctors were all smiles.

As we are about to leave, instead of saying goodbye to Dr. Catevenis, I say "hello." He instantly remembers that as the first word I said when I emerged from my coma. He grins and nods proudly.

When we get home that night, my mom reminds me what Dr. Daee told us: I must stay off my feet and relax as much as possible, which means that I won't be going to physical therapy for at least a week.

I take this period to work on my art. Ever since I was a young child, I would draw, color, sketch, and paint—anywhere and on anything. That was how I expressed my emotions. Because I don't have any memory of the accident and can only recall hazy, disjointed periods from when I was in the coma, I want to see if I'm able to pry loose these hidden, repressed memories through art. Perhaps through this self-expression, I will find deeply buried answers that have been eluding me.

There was no sense of time when I was comatose. Randomness was the mental ordering principle as my body was mechanically kept alive. Unmoored from reality, my mind naturally played tricks. To illustrate this hallucinatory period, I use symbolic colors and images, disorienting compositions of blurred first-person perspectives. The use of black and white delineates a shifting boundary between life and death, while red represents the medium connecting both states.

When I start drawing, I don't have a fixed idea in place but simply allow the subconscious to guide my hand. The most amazing thing happens: memory fragments push their way to the surface, which I transform into a visually symbolic representation. These images then tell my story, decipherable to no one but myself.

I call this drawing "Time is of the Essence":

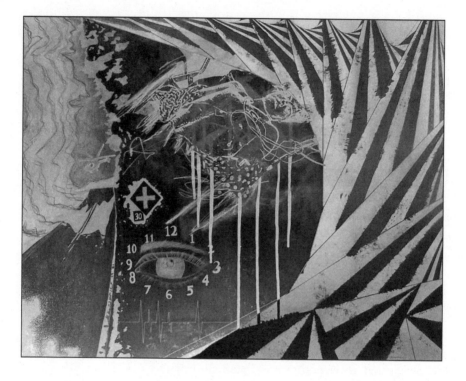

After a week of bed rest, I'm anxious to return to the school track to continue walking and jogging. But what I most want to do is get in the pool. After several conversations with my family practice doctor, Jaleh Daee, who is the wife of my main surgeon, we decide that I must first pass two physical tests—a chest X-ray and pulmonary exam for repiratory function—before getting my toes wet. She says that my healing is incomplete and I must wait another month.

Two days before Christmas, both test results come back positive. Later the same day, my parents and I head over to the nearby Henry

E. Lackey high school aquatic center. The last time I was here was on July 6, the day of the accident.

The pool is crowded, but I find an open lane. I'm wearing the swimsuit and goggles that the St. Mary's swim team gave me. I stand at the edge of the pool and look down into the water. My father is filming me with a DVD camera. I'm actually nervous—will I sink or swim? I notice several pairs of eyes staring at all the scars on my shoulders, chest, and stomach. Despite my discomfort at the gawking, I want to give these people a show.

I would prefer to dive into the water, but my balance is still shaky. So I lean over and fall into the pool. I plummet right to the bottom, but I have no intention of immediately surfacing. The sensation is too wonderful. I feel both weightless and free from all pain.

After about fifteen seconds, I push off the pool bottom with my feet. When I surface, I begin to tread water, something I wasn't sure I would be able to do. I look over at my parents who are clapping their hands, smiling. I slowly lift my right arm a few inches above the water and use my left arm to scull beneath my body to support my weight, which slightly propels me forward. I repeat the movement, while lowering my head into the water and giving a few easy flutter kicks with my feet. Then it happens—I'm swimming! Once again, the impossible has been made possible. My body moves through the water, while I partially lift my head to breathe on the left and then right. My arms knife through the water. It's not some aquatic magic trick that I am performing; there are no illusions. This is real and it is beautiful, a defiance of doubters and physical limitations.

I swim halfway across the pool, then stop to hang onto the lane rope and catch my breath. I swim back to the wall and take another rest.

I repeat this several times until I feel ready for my first lap. I kick off from the wall and begin swimming. When I make it to the other end, I'm winded. My damaged left shoulder aches and I hold on to the edge of the pool.

It takes the remainder of my dwindling strength to climb out of the pool. After a quick shower in the men's locker room, I walk back out on the pool deck to meet my parents. We leave the pool center laughing and in great spirits. The last time I exited these doors, I was on my way to an unanticipated appointment with a dump truck.

I return to the pool later in the week with my good buddy Sam Fleming, who is a year younger than me. He went to a rival high school and swam the fifty-meter breaststroke. He was fast, really fast. We first met at an afternoon practice at my summer league pool. He was quiet with a tenacious attitude. Even though he's currently in the middle of a competitive swim season, he wants to help out as my new coach.

We spend most of our time treading water and doing light strength-training exercises on the pool deck. We follow this routine for weeks, and slowly but surely, I build the stamina to swim continuous laps. We don't stop there—in time, we train five days a week. We work out with weights at the local college, including a mixture of plyometrics, stretching, and slow running.

All of this sounds unbelievable. I have become a swimmer again, despite everything that conspired against me. With my still-damaged lungs and the ever-present pain in my left shoulder, I'm much slower in the water than I used to be. But I don't mind, because when my body is in the pool, I am moving. That is what really counts. Not too long ago, I was motionless, strapped down in a hospital bed. When I'm swimming, I feel like the freest person on the planet.

CHAPTER 24

TATTOOS

ONE MORNING AS I'M LOOKING IN THE MIRROR AT THE MANY SCARS decorating my left arm and shoulder, I think it's time to do something creative: get a tattoo. It won't be my first. When I was fifteen, I got a lightning bolt tattoo on my right shoulder. The bolt symbolized victory and the unpredictability of life. It suited my fierce competitive drive in sports.

So, on my nineteenth birthday, about ten months after the accident, I decide on a second tattoo to commemorate my new victory in life and to celebrate a birthday that I almost didn't have. This tattoo is the Greek word "alpha" and would be inked on my left shoulder, over traces of shattered glass and black paint from the car that infused itself into my scarred flesh.

"Alpha" was the classification of my status when I arrived at the hospital by medevac. For shock trauma victims, alpha signifies the absolute worst for the victim, who is usually minutes from death. In most cases, that means the patient could be dead on arrival.

Dr. James Catevenis, the codirector of the Intensive Care Unit at Prince George's Hospital, is Greek, and the tattoo would also serve as a permanent tribute to him. For over two months, he did his best to make sure that I would live to see another day.

My Uncle Joe drives me to a tattoo parlor in Waldorf, Maryland, called the Blue Scarab. Because my left shoulder is the side where I was hit by the dump truck, the tattoo artist has to work around the scarred flesh still embedded with small pieces of broken glass and black paint fragments from the Camaro.

CHAPTER 25

CONCRETE

LATE SPRING 2005. NOT QUITE A YEAR SINCE THE ACCIDENT. MY DAYS are now spent around concrete. Lots of it. I like going to work with my dad. Every morning, I wake up around five in the morning and think what a great privilege it is to easily slide my legs from under the blanket and over the side of the bed onto the floor. Breakfast is usually a bowl of Lucky Charms with milk and a glass of orange juice. Then it's out the door and into my dad's truck for our thirty-minute drive to where his concrete pump truck is stationed.

A concrete pump truck is not the same as those barrel-shaped ready-mix trucks one sees on roads or at construction sites. Because most work sites are often crowded with machinery and building materials, the process of pouring concrete can be challenging. The concrete pump truck allows one to get close to where fresh concrete needs to be poured. The pump operator uses a radio-controlled device to position the boom pipeline into the desired area to be filled. The boom itself is a mechanical arm that extends from the truck and is made up of a long series of pipes through which the concrete flows, and can range from fifty-six to two hundred feet in length. The concrete moves through the pipes via a hydraulic networking system. My dad's pump truck is capable of 105 feet, which is sufficient for a wide assortment of jobs—housing foundation slabs, driveways, swimming pools, as well as commercial and industrial projects. A typical workday can range between ten and fourteen hours, and might have us going out to six different sites.

The concrete itself is brought in from ready-mix trucks that back up to the receiving end of the pump truck called the hopper, which then sends the concrete through the boom and out the hose at the other end. Most people think that concrete and cement are the same thing because the words are often used interchangeably, but cement is actually one of the ingredients of concrete, along with sand and gravel.

For the first few weeks, I mostly do maintenance tasks such as cleaning and waxing the truck, making sure to remove all the concrete fragments before they dry and chip the paint, shining the chrome on the wheels and wiping the tires with Armor All, and cleaning the windows. It's tiring work, but my left shoulder and arm benefit from the physical activity. I soon progress to lifting heavy two-by-fours and concrete blocks. The more I lift, the stronger I get. By the end of spring, my weight is back up to 180 pounds. Another bonus: by wearing construction boots usually covered in concrete, my legs also get a terrific daily workout.

On slower days, Dad lets me set up the truck. It's an adrenaline rush to operate a machine that costs $500,000. But I must always remain extra careful. So many things can go wrong. Over the years, my dad has personally witnessed many accidents on job sites. On a medium-rise commercial building project in Tysons Corner, Virginia, a guy on the open third floor was using an air compressor to blow away debris. He slipped off the edge and landed on a one-inch-thick iron rod that punctured his stomach. Even though he was in shock, a coworker handed him a cigarette, which he partially smoked, while waiting for the rescue workers to come and saw off the rod before rushing him to the hospital for emergency surgery.

Another time, my dad was working at Union Station in Washington, D.C., when a coworker was on top of the dome replacing sheet metal. The worker's safety–restraint belt broke and he slid down fifty feet, with the metal's sharp jagged ends shredding his body. A two-foot-wide water gutter stopped his fall. He ended up in critical condition.

On another occasion when my dad was working at a parking garage at Georgetown University, a guy on the second floor was stripping away metal wall forms with a thirty-pound iron-digging bar. The bar slipped through his hands and fell to the lower level where it hit a coworker, smashing his hard hat into pieces and cracking his skull. He was killed instantly.

The reason he tells me these stories is not to frighten me, but because he wants me to understand just how dangerous the construction industry is. Yet in the thirty-five years that he has worked in this business, he has never had any safety problems or caused any injuries. He has trained thirty pump-truck operators, always telling them that anybody can run a pump truck, but to be a successful operator, you have to be a successful troubleshooter. His stellar safety record verifies that statement many times over.

When I get home from work, I usually head to the local rec pool. All the construction work has strengthened me. I can swim longer and faster. On some days, I meet Sam at the pool or the gym to lift weights. I continue working with my dad right through the summer. We decide that I should attend St. Mary's College in the fall. Sam will be my roommate in one of the dorms. We will also be teammates on the swim team. A year ago, all of this would have seemed highly unlikely. No, make that impossible, even insane, to consider college and actually being on the swim team. I still have difficulty wrapping my mind around how I outfoxed death and survived a coma, paralysis, seizures, and infections. I am grateful for each and every day.

CHAPTER 26

ST. MARY'S COLLEGE SWIM TEAM

IT'S HARD TO BELIEVE THAT I AM FINALLY HERE—AT ST MARY'S. THE beautiful campus sits next to the St. Mary's River. The school was established in 1840 and academic pursuits are a priority here. It's a small school, with about two thousand students. St. Mary's City was the fourth outpost of colonization in British North America and was the capital of Maryland until 1695.

After unloading all my stuff into my room and saying goodbye to my parents, Sam and I check out the college's new fifty-meter pool. I'm amazed by its sheer size and try to calculate how many gallons of water went into filling it up. I visualize the pool being filled with millions of my teardrops, because that is exactly what it took for me to get here.

We have a week of classes before our first swim practice. All the guys and the girls on the team are like a small family, which I definitely prefer since I'm incredibly self-conscious walking around with my visible scars. My local rec pool was dimly lit and rarely crowded. However, the lights inside the new St. Mary's aquatic center are bright. You can see every red and pink scar on my body, which makes me want to walk around with a shirt on, or at least have a towel draped over my shoulders.

Because I was introduced to the team at a preseason meeting, the other swimmers already know about the accident. But this is the first occasion that they have seen me without a shirt, so the questions begin flying immediately, though not in an uncomfortable way. I keep my answers short and as upbeat as possible, providing a condensed version of the events.

When it's time to swim, I go hard and strong with the rest of the sprinters. But after thirty minutes, my body begins shutting down. I try to push through the fatigue and stay focused, but exhaustion wins. I stroke to the side of the pool, feeling cramps in my legs, arms, and neck. A sympathetic and supportive Coach Barbins walks over to see if I'm okay. I say that I just need a quick drink and then I'll be good.

I take some sips from my water bottle, then get the drive to continue on through the pain. I kick off the wall triumphantly and achieve a nice rhythm with the other swimmers. I don't want anyone to think that I'm unable to keep up with the pace, especially on the first day when everyone is checking out one another. The last thing I want is my teammates to feel sorry for me, grant me favors, or think that I'm not good enough to be on the team. But my body can take only so much. After another fifteen minutes, I head to the pool edge and remove my swim cap and goggles. I feel dejected and vulnerable, as if I've just let everyone down, especially myself.

I collect my kickboard, water bottle, and pull buoy and climb out of the pool. I toss the kickboard and pull buoy in the metal bin and walk alone to the locker room with my head down in shame, unwilling to look up at any of the swimmers in the pool.

It's time for a serious reality check while I take a shower. The hot water can't remove the obvious: I was an idiot to think that I could swim at this elite level. Everyone is much faster than me. I can't even make it through *half* a practice. This is a big mistake. So why beat myself up over my physical limitations? My teammates weren't crushed by a truck; they didn't have their organs shattered and body battered. When I was fighting for my life fourteen months ago, they were able to stay fit and swim whenever they wanted, living healthy normal lives. While I was learning how to walk and take a piss without any help, they were deep in training.

Yet if I overcame death, why have I become such a defeatist simply because I can't swim hard for an hour? Now is *not* the time to quit. If I give up, it's not because I can't do it, it's because I *think* I can't do it. I turn off the shower and decide to show up for swim practice tomorrow. I can do this.

The next day I get back in the pool with the team. I'm doing the best that I can and that's all I can hope to achieve. I swim hard for forty-five minutes and then get out of the pool. And this is how it goes for the remainder of the first week. I attend classes, do homework, and go to swim practice. It's a good routine. I call my parents after every practice to give them an update on how everything is going with school and in the pool. They are pleased to hear from me.

The next week, I speak with Coach Barbins. We decide that I should swim two or three times a week instead of six like everyone else. It's not that I'm incapable of swimming every day, but there's a concern that my heart and lungs need the extra days of rest. We want to stay on the prudent side of caution.

I also decide to move out of the dorm and live at home. I will commute to school instead of staying on campus. I think it's too early for my parents to be alone after everything we went through over the past year. After spending practically every waking minute with them and experiencing so many hardships together, I find that it's emotionally hard on them for me to just disappear into college life. My mom tells me that when I'm not around, my dad becomes quiet and mopes around the house like a lost dog.

On the days when I don't swim, I lift weights and run on the treadmill to keep up my conditioning. My left shoulder is still not 100 percent; there's still nerve damage. My lungs haven't flushed out all the junk and liquid. I can't jump more than a few inches off the ground because my ankles are weak. This matters in swim races because you need sufficient ankle strength to spring off the starting block and push off the walls.

With a little over two months of training under our Speedos, we're ready for our first swim meet with Hood College, which will be held in the new aquatic center. Because Coach Barbins knows how badly I want to swim in this meet, he gives me the privilege of swimming in the two-hundred-yard medley relay team, which is the first event.

On November 11, 2005, I walk out into the center with the rest of the St. Mary's Seahawks swim team. We're wearing our school colors—navy blue, yellow gold, and white. My parents are watching in the crowded bleachers. The announcer introduces the first race.

I take off my blue team parka and set it down on a bench. I instantly sense stares from the people in the stands, the timing officials, and especially the opposing team. I hear people whispering, and I know what they're saying, but my still-visible scars, I realize, are the triumphant symbol of loving life. These scars are my proud battle wounds.

I put on my goggles and swim cap, then head over to the designated starting blocks with the other swimmers. Sam is a few lanes down from me, swinging his arms to get loose. He sees me and gives a thumbs-up. Each school has two relay teams, and mine is in lane one.

In the two-hundred-yard medley relay, each swimmer goes two laps. The four events, in order, are backstroke, butterfly, breaststroke, and freestyle. I'm swimming the freestyle, which means that I'm the anchor leg.

When the race official says, "Judges and timers ready," my body suddenly grows weak. However, "swimmers take their marks" snaps me back into reality. Then *beep*!

As the swimmers blast across the pool, I focus on what I must do. Two of the other relay teams have a lap lead when my breaststroking teammate is about fifteen feet from the wall. He is neck and neck with the swimmer in the adjacent lane. It will be a race for third place.

I rapidly inhale and exhale several times, trying to remove all the lingering carbon dioxide so only fresh oxygen remains in my lungs.

Ten feet.

I swing my arms in a circle for that final stretch and press my goggles tightly against my eyes.

Five feet.

I crouch so my hands are near my feet, and my fingers grip the edge of the starting block.

Three . . . two . . . one, and my teammate's fingers touches the wall.

I leap off the block, kicking hard to glide those extra feet underwater. When I surface, I'm churning though the water at full-throttle, maintaining proper form and technique. Before I know it, I'm already doing a flip turn at the wall. The swimmer to my left won't back down.

I really put the steam on, giving everything I have. My lungs are on fire and I refuse to take any more breaths. I dig down deep to block the lactic-acid pain. I elongate my stroke. I'm only a few yards away from the wall when I notice that he's starting to fall back. But I can't take the risk of him charging for the wall at the last second. The black line at the pool bottom has changed into a fuzzy dark line as exhaustion overwhelms me. My arms feel heavy, like they're not joined to my body. I push harder. Several more feet and I'm there. I slam my hand so hard against the wall that a wave of water splashes up out of the pool and drenches the timing official.

Our relay team takes third. My individual split is around twenty-four seconds, only a second slower than my personal record in high school. I give high fives to my teammates, but they're wondering why I'm excited about third place. Need I remind them that doctors and physical therapists once thought I would never be able to swim again? To me, third place is as good as gold.

I run up to the bleachers and give my parents a big old hug. But I have to hurry back down to the pool deck because I have one more event to swim—the individual fifty-yard freestyle.

I'm back on the starting block. I hear the beep and race through the two laps in roughly the same time as before—twenty-four seconds. It earns a fourth place out of eight swimmers.

BY THE END OF THE FALL SEMESTER, I'VE RACED IN THREE MORE SWIM meets. For Christmas, my parents surprise me with the ultimate gift—they are going to build a pool in the backyard. BRIAN'S POOL is scribbled in blue colored pencil at the bottom of the blueprints. It will be ready by early summer. But during winter break, I get sick again. Excess fluid has built up in my lungs. I come down with bronchitis and early-onset mononucleosis. The most likely culprit for this health setback is a compromised immune system due to swim training; my body's natural resistance to infections is still low. Regretfully, I'm forced to stop swimming. Instead, I will spend more time lifting weights to build back my strength.

So while I attend classes at St. Mary's, I find an athletic outlet with my old love: weight training. It's certainly not a team sport—just me and the heavy iron. Yet I have no complaints because I'm gradually getting stronger and healthier. That's what's really at stake here: I must convince others as well as myself that I have the desire, ability, and means to be the athlete that everyone once knew me as. I can't make those endless days and nights in the hospital vanish. What I can do is make people not focus on that bleak period whenever they see me. Each day then becomes a slow, methodical, and deliberate movement toward reaching my goal to become fit. By early summer, with classes out, I start to feel much better about my appearance and myself. Muscles certainly help my self-esteem as well as warding off depression.

CHAPTER 27

JULY IS THE CRUELEST MONTH

GOD MUST HAVE A MORBID SENSE OF HUMOR. OR LIFE IS SIMPLY FILLED with unexplained mysteries and uncanny coincidences. Take your pick: destiny, luck, or fate? Or all three?

As the accident's second anniversary approaches, I can't help but feel the obsessive need to relive the day's events—a day I don't even remember, and which I've only been able to reconstruct from what my parents and others have told me. I'm not looking forward to July 6. It's like I should hold an anti-celebration to permanently place that day forever behind me.

On the day before, July 5, 2006, as I'm finishing up a weight-lifting workout at home, I get a call from my dad. "Brian, something bad has happened to Nana. She's in the hospital."

"Why? What's wrong?"

"She was at the doctor's earlier this afternoon and they ended up rushing her to the hospital."

My grandmother's health has been declining for some time. She's been out in and out of the hospital several times. Her latest health scare resulted in quadruple bypass surgery several years ago.

I'm very close to Nana, my mother's mother. She's a classy, glamorous lady who always had her hair and nails done. But she was also the type of person who wasn't afraid to kick off her shoes and play soccer or hockey with me in the basement. Or, we'd go to the lake to fish, dribble a basketball around, draw together, or even watch cartoons on the television. She was always fun to be around and told great stories. A great buddy.

When my parents and I arrive at the hospital, we are directed to Intensive Care. Uh-oh, I know what this means. We see my grandfather, Big D, first. He's wearing sunglasses to hide his tears. I've never seen him like this before. He looks shaken, dazed, even shocked.

We find out from my Uncle Joe that she's in a coma. When I hear that word—*coma*—I'm overwhelmed by vivid flashbacks. Walking into her room is like stepping into the past. The same beeping and pinging machines that kept me alive are keeping Nana alive. She's lying in bed, unresponsive and motionless, connected to a nest of tubes. Her eyes are closed but then sporadically flicker open from either the medication or irregular electrical nerve impulses misfiring in her brain. A ventilator is doing her breathing. A nurse dabs Nana's forehead with a damp cloth. My heart is breaking as I stand by her bed. The nurse says that she went into cardiac arrest earlier in the day before slipping into a coma.

Throughout the rest of the afternoon and evening, I repeatedly go in to check on her between visits from other family members, and see if I can get any responses from her by slightly squeezing her hand. I know what it's like to be trapped inside a locked-in body and how you need to make a connection to the outside world. But Nana barely responds to my touch.

I return to the hospital the next morning with my parents. Holding her limp hand, I tearfully read her a letter that I composed a few hours before. I don't know if she can hear or understand me. I'm an emotional wreck when I get to the end.

One week later, she passes away.

CHAPTER 28

BODYBUILDING

Over the years, I have collected several pieces of exercise equipment, including a treadmill, stationary bike, bench-press system with a leg device to work the hamstrings and quadriceps, and an inexpensive Nautilus machine. I also have a punching bag, barbells, and set of dumbbells. I prefer to work out with free weights because it allows you to control the weight throughout the various movements.

When I swam in high school, I needed to be lean, so I lifted light weights for repetition to build muscular endurance. But when it was time to bulk up for throwing the discus in track season, I switched my focus to lifting heavier weight at low repetitions. Now that my collegiate swimming career is on standby, I decide to concentrate on building muscle bulk. When I get home from classes at St. Mary's, I eat dinner, do homework, and then work out for an hour and fifteen minutes. I often add some cardio on the treadmill.

Within several weeks, I've gained a noticeable amount of weight. My diet consists of a protein shake at breakfast with two cups of oatmeal and a glass of orange juice. For lunch, it's a turkey sandwich on whole wheat bread, a granola bar, a banana, another protein shake, and some yogurt.

For dinner, I eat two chicken breasts, or lean meat and rice, or fish with a vegetable. For dessert, it's another protein shake. Between the meals, I continually have healthy snacks—rice cakes, celery, carrots, peanuts, cashews, and apples.

By mid-May, I've gained about twenty pounds, which finally puts me up to about two hundred pounds—a weight gain of seventy pounds since I left Intensive Care twenty months ago. I also feel better about my physical appearance because the scars on my stomach, arms, neck, and chest have started to fade from a garish blood-red to a more tolerable light pink. My left shoulder is improving as well, but it still gives me trouble on the bench press.

The bench press has always been my favorite exercise. My interest started back in sixth grade when I began lifting on a bench press in our garage. As I became older, I bench-pressed heavier weights; I never really had formal training, but in my junior year in high school, I entered a regional power-lifting championship and competed in the 181-pound division. I took first place.

I've always wanted to pursue amateur bodybuilding. Like many others in the sport, I'm a big fan of Arnold Schwarzenegger, especially after seeing the classic 1970s bodybuilding documentary "Pumping Iron." Another world-class bodybuilder I follow is Jay Cutler, a two-time Mr. Olympia winner who now lives in Las Vegas. Many think Jay's the next Arnold. I've read his magazine profiles, researched his background, and kept up-to-date on all his important wins. He stands only five feet nine, but his massive arms are twenty-one inches and his bulging chest measures fifty-six inches.

One day as I'm looking at Jay's website, I send him a quick email to introduce myself and see if he can offer any advice. The next day, he fires off an email to me with helpful workout tips—daily exercise routines, when to rest, how much cardio I should be getting, and proper foods to gain lean muscle. Later, he sends me an autographed copy of his book, several workout DVDs, shirts, and a cap.

Following his recommendations, my revised workout program consists of upper-body routines on Mondays, Wednesdays, and Fridays. The lower-body routines take place on Tuesdays, Thursdays, and Saturdays. On each day, I usually do about three sets of ten different exercises, starting with eight reps, then six reps, followed by four reps. On Sunday, I take a break from all training and allow my muscles to recover.

I log every single workout in a grade-school composition book. It doesn't take long to see noticeable results on paper and in the mirror. It seems like only yesterday I was bench-pressing a broomstick in the large physical therapy room at Kernan Rehabilitation Center, and now I'm able to lift 225 pounds for a single maximum effort. Back then, I struggled to bicep-curl two and a half pounds, and now I'm up to thirty pounds. Best of all, a Canadian nutritional supplement company that manufactures whey protein powder called 4EverFit, as well as selling a wide range of products for hard-core bodybuilders, has contacted me in regard to sponsoring my amateur bodybuilding career.

I have all the motivation in the world to see how far I can take my bodybuilding. By Christmas, I weigh 240 pounds. Two years ago, in 2004, I was a fraction of this size, weak, feeble, and uncertain about whether any of my withered muscles would reappear. I had just graduated from a wheelchair imprisonment. Now I can bench-press 375 pounds and bicep-curl 50 pounds. I've had to buy an entire new wardrobe. My friends and parents are amazed by my physical transformation. I can't help but laugh when I think about what it would be like to swim in this kind of bulked-up shape. Yet when I look in the mirror and do bodybuilding poses, I don't always see beefcake Brian staring back. I see instead sickly Brian on life support in Intensive Care. Even though I look larger in the reflection, I feel diminished and frail. My mind remains in a state of denial, unwilling to accept my radical body makeover. No matter how many new pounds of muscle I've managed to accumulate, I still see an emaciated victim underneath muscle-plated armor. Nonetheless, as a reminder of how far I traveled on the road to recovery, I keep a photo by my bed that was taken shortly after leaving Intensive Care: I'm sitting in the wheelchair, slumped over with my hands folded and head lowered. This sad, forlorn image that signifies defeat always makes me nervous that the moment I stop working out, all the progress I've made can be stripped away. Because my life before and after the accident remains joined together as dueling realities, I am always aware of how lucky I was to escape death, and escape being permanently trapped in a non-functioning body. The effort of taking a shower, for example, is a daily reminder that my scars are as much mental as physical. The bodybuilding pushes me forward, allowing a positive reawakening of my athletic potential.

That is why I constantly remind myself to live in the present even though the post-accident phase demands to ride shotgun. During that first month home from Intensive Care, Dad had to carry me upstairs so he and my mom could bathe me just like when I was little. He even joked, "Don't forget you're probably going to have to do this for me in twenty years." He actually believed that I'd be healthy and normal again one day. After every shower, he'd carry me to my bed where I'd sit in my bathrobe and look at my thin reflection in the mirror and ask myself repeatedly: *Is this really me?*

But now, the *new* me is the one who worked hard and long for the past year to pack on weight and muscles because that is my real identity—not Skeleton Boy.

THROUGH MY WEIGHT TRAINING AND BODYBUILDING OVER THE PAST year, I've learned a lot about fitness and nutrition. I consider getting a part-time job as a personal trainer. My athletic background and recovery from the accident will help people achieve their fitness-related goals. Look how far I've come since the crash. Glancing back, however, those two years seemed endless because the recovery took place in small, everyday increments. There were no shortcuts.

To become certified as a personal trainer, I first needed to pass a test, There are several types of exams for certification, but the one usually recommended is from the American Council of Exercise. The nearby College of Southern Maryland offers this test, so I invest in a thick textbook and study manual. A lot of the material deals with anatomy, some of which I learned throughout my rehab—bones, muscles, joints, and ligaments. Then there's exercise physiology and how it relates to a potential client's age and health. After studying for several weeks, I take the three-hour test that features 150 multiple choice questions as well as a written simulation test with two client scenarios.

Because I won't know my test results for at least a month, I find an entry-level job at the Sport & Health Club where I started working out after I came home from the hospital with my Uncle Joe. Members range in age from teens to senior citizens. Most of the women work out on the upper level with the resistance equipment, elliptical machines, treadmills, and stationary bikes. The guys mainly work out downstairs with bench presses, leg press machines, squat racks, and free weights.

My tasks entail going around with paper towels and a disinfectant spray bottle to clean the equipment and shadow other personal trainers. I like walking around in my red T-shirt with the club logo, answering members' questions about the exercise machines.

After a month of working at the gym, I receive a letter in the mail from the American Council of Exercise. I open the white envelope in the driveway, look at my test scores, and see that it says CONGRATULATIONS in big bold letters at the bottom of the page listing my passing score. I drive back to the gym to proudly show my bosses the official documentation that I'm certified and can begin finding and training clients.

My first client is Kawanda, who is a military mother in her mid-thirties and slightly overweight. I have talked to her on several occasions in the gym. She knows about my background with the accident and recovery, and I think that is why she wants me as her personal trainer. She knows that I understand the frustration of being out of shape and the desire to get healthy and fit.

Kawanda's most pressing concern is passing the U.S. Army's annual physical training test. One requirement is running one and a half miles. She says that her running is weak. For our first session, I start her out with some light stretching for about five minutes and then we go over to the treadmill for ten minutes to get her muscles activated. Then we do thirty minutes of light strength-training routines on the various machines. In addition to toning and conditioning exercises, I recommend that she join a group fitness or spinning class. Our session ends with several minutes on the stationary bike for a cool down. We decide that I will be her personal trainer on Mondays, Wednesdays, and Fridays.

My second client is a middle-aged mother named Karen who is trying to lose the weight she gained during her recent pregnancy. I help design a plan that will also improve her overall conditioning level because she used to be active before she became pregnant. We're scheduled to meet three times a week.

My third client is Aaryn, who is a collegiate swimmer and wants help with her strength training. I put together a fairly hard-core plan that focuses on shoulders, core strength, and leg power. I recommend that she do two sessions a week with me.

Outside of personal training, I'm also teaching swim lessons during the week to a high school sophomore swimmer named Rachel. She's been swimming competitively for several years and wants extra help with the one-hundred-yard butterfly. We drive to a local pool to practice for an hour. I usually have her do one-arm drills, swimming with a resistance band, and swimming at race pace.

Because of the amount of time I was required to spend in physical therapy after my long hospitalization, I feel like I have a unique perspective in helping my nonathletic clients. It's a wonderful motivational tool— even for myself when I occasionally imagine that I'm back in the hospital. I know I must live in the present, but the past is something I can't seem to escape from either.

PART THREE

SOUL

CHAPTER 29

MY FIRST TRIATHLON

Before the accident severely rearranged my future in sports, I toyed with the idea of someday competing in an Ironman triathlon—a 2.4-mile swim, 112-mile bike ride, and 26.2-mile run. The granddaddy of the Ironman is in Kona, Hawaii. I watched the Hawaii Ironman on television, and was always fascinated by those who competed in the world's toughest single-day endurance race.

My unfortunate encounter with the dump truck, however, shelved those Iron dreams. They naturally turned to rust. Even when I was sufficiently recovered and swimming and lifting weights, the Ironman seemed an impossible quest, on par with winning the Powerball lottery. Yet on a whim one afternoon, almost three years since the crash, I decide to check out the Ironman website. *Perhaps in several years*, I fantasize, *I might be physically ready to participate in an Ironman triathlon.*

The Ironman's motto is "Anything is possible." I can certainly relate to that phrase. I notice on the website that there's a "contact us" button, so I begin typing an email seeking information about how to register for a race. But then I get emotionally carried away and allow the words to gush out. I tell them all the details of my accident, trauma, and recovery.

ABOUT SIX WEEKS LATER, WHILE I'M ON THE COMPUTER AND LISTENING to Ted Nugent's "Stranglehold," Peter Henning of the Ironman sends me an email.

Dear Brian,

I am the producer of the NBC television show for the Ironman. Your story is certainly worthy of being a feature story on the NBC show. Have you been participating in any triathlons? If so, please send me a list of the races and how you did. Where have you been training for the Ironman? I would like to speak with you in person. If all the criteria are met, and I don't see why they wouldn't be, we definitely would like to follow your day in Kona and video an interview at your home, and also shoot some training on the bike and run. Do you still live near the hospital that treated you? If so, are any of the doctors who worked on you still at that hospital? I am also sure our PR/ Media department would like to get involved as well.

I immediately call Peter, but judging from his initial questions, I assume he thinks I'm still in a wheelchair. I explain that I've recovered quite a bit since I was let out of the hospital and tell him about my bodybuilding. So he knows that I'm fit. But I'm in no shape to do a triathlon. The longest swim race I would normally do on the swim team was a hundred yards. The ocean swim in the Ironman covers 2.4 miles— that's equivalent to just over forty-two hundred-yard races. It's also been years since I've been on a bicycle. And running is something I usually do on a treadmill for ten or fifteen minutes. How could I possibly get in shape for the 2007 Hawaii Ironman that was less than four months away? This is a race that requires a year of serious training, and that's assuming you're already in decent shape. While I can lift a small mountain of iron at the gym, I'm far from being an aerobic warrior. I have the muscles, not the cardio. I'd be a disaster, a total train wreck in a triathlon.

Peter reassures me that after all I've been through, I won't have trouble with the mental aspect of the race. But he emphasizes that since I have never done a triathlon, I have to prove to him that I'm physically capable of swimming, biking, and running for a full day. Most importantly, the first thing I need to do is to get my doctors' medical approval. If I receive a thumbs-up from all of them, says Peter, then the next step is to complete a half-Ironman triathlon, which consists of a 1.2-mile swim, 56-mile bike ride, and 13.1-mile run. I must be able to finish this race without any medical problems and within the required time limit. Once these two steps are completed, the NBC staff in charge of the Ironman broadcast will decide whether I will get a media slot to compete in the Hawaii Ironman in Kona on October 13.

I tell him that I'm interested and will get the ball rolling by talking to my doctors. When I hang up, I'm bouncing off the walls with excitement. I call my mom at work to tell her the big news, but I detect hesitation and noticeable tension in her voice. "Uh . . . the Hawaii Ironman? The race we always watch on TV? That Hawaii Ironman? When is it?" The protective motherly instinct takes over.

"In October," I respond

"No, Brian, come on, that's crazy. It's mid-July, There's no way you'll have enough time to train for a race in October. Can you ask them if you can do it next year? Your body's not even completely healed." Her voice is full of panic.

This isn't the response I expected, but I do agree with her about the timing. October is awfully close and I'm definitely not ready for something like this—but how can I pass up this opportunity? I call my dad next.

"Hey Dad, guess what?" I say cheerfully, hoping that he hasn't already talked to my mom. I tell him the good news.

"What? Are you kidding? That's fantastic! That's the big triathlon, too. When is it? And what did your mom say?"

He agrees with her that it's too soon, and then there's the issue of my lack of training. He suggests that we should have a family discussion when everyone is home.

While I wait for them, I sit down in a reclining chair by our newly built pool and review my prospects. I don't own one of those fancy triathlon bikes. The most biking I've ever done was on a cheap recreational bike when I was younger. I've done no open-water swimming. And running? Even though I was on my high school track team, the most I ran was from the throwing circle out to fetch the shot put or discus. I'm not even sure how one is supposed to train for a triathlon. Plus I feel sluggish from all the weight that I've gained as a bodybuilder. For the past year and a half, I have not been doing much cardio because I have focused on lifting heavy weights. All this accumulated muscle mass is now my enemy in a triathlon. From what I've seen on the Ironman telecast and on their website, there aren't many triathletes who weigh 230 pounds. I need to lay off the protein powders and six meals a day. If I can lose a few pounds before the half-Ironman race, then I'll be lighter on my feet. But my main concern is obtaining the medical approvals. And for that to happen, I first need my parents' permission.

After my dad gets home, I stand by the front door and look out the window as I watch my mom drive down the driveway and pull into the garage. I think about all the words that I've mentally rehearsed, but as soon as she opens the door, my mind goes blank.

"Hey Mom, how was your day?"

She puts her hand up and stops me short. "I have no problem with you doing the Ironman next year. But this year is way too soon."

Later that night after dinner, I spell it all out for her. "Mom, I understand exactly how you feel and I don't blame you. But when has something this great happened to me? It's a like a gift. If I can do this race, it's going to show that I'm healthy, and I need to know that, because I still feel like I have to hold back in life, that I have limitations and restraints on what I can and can't physically do. Every time I cough or sneeze, you want to rush me to the hospital. We need to know that my body is healthy and normal again, and if I can finish this race, that will be our answer."

She doesn't buy my argument. In fact, she has that same anxious look that I was used to seeing in my hospital room, but this time she stands her ground and doesn't duck out of sight. "Brian, you've never done a triathlon. Where are you going to get the bike and gear? We're still paying off our medical bills. I'm concerned about your health. I don't know if your heart and lungs could even handle this. You could die out there— have you thought about that?"

"Mom, if the doctors don't give me a medical clearance, then I won't do it. I'll thank Mr. Henning for his time and interest and I'll never bring it up to you again. But let's just see what the doctors have to say before we shoot the entire idea down."

My dad chimes in. "JoAnne, look at what he's been able to do. He has defied the odds over and over. Brian has never failed at anything that he has put his mind to. I believe that he can do this."

She finally relents. "Well, I think hearing from your doctors will help me feel better."

THE NEXT DAY, SHE SPEAKS WITH DR. DAEE, WHO IS FAMILIAR WITH THE Ironman. He believes that I will be fine doing the race, though he suggests that I meet with my cardiologist, Dr. Saeed Koolaee, for his opinion. Dr. Daee's preliminary green light gives me hope. After all, he operated on my vital organs several times.

The next doctor on our list is Dr. Catevenis, so my parents and I drive up to Prince George's Hospital and we ask him what he thinks about the race. Dr. Boyce, the ICU codirector, is also there. They both tell me they are fine with me doing the race as long as I promise them that I will take my time and that if I feel any possible trouble with my heart rate or breathing abilities, I'll take a break or quit.

The following week, I schedule an appointment with Dr. James Harring, who is our family doctor and is familiar with my hospitalization and recovery. He doesn't think that I should have many problems with the Ironman as long as I pace myself and don't overdo it. He takes some blood samples before I leave.

The final person to see is Dr. Koolaee, who will be the deciding factor. My mom comes with me. She wants to hear his thoughts about the Ironman, because, for one thing, I might be on the course for up to seventeen hours.

The last time Dr. Koolaee saw me, I had just been released from the hospital and was in a wheelchair and extremely thin. He is surprised by how much progress I've made.

He begins the checkup by taking my blood pressure. "Well, your blood pressure looks good. Any problems with your heart rate in the past few months? Like when you work out with weights, or swim?" He places his hand around my wrist to measure my pulse.

"Well, to be honest, I try to focus on listening to my body, especially my heart, when I'm doing any type of physical exercise," I respond. "I haven't had any problems since that second scare when I went back to the hospital for five days. I've been okay since then."

He takes his stethoscope and listens to my chest and back. "Your heart rate looks normal too, but I still want to run a series of echocardiography tests on your heart." We schedule the tests for Saturday.

FOR THE REST OF THE WEEK, I CAN'T GO FIVE MINUTES WITHOUT THINKING about the tests. Saturday finally arrives and my parents and I make the trip to Dr. Koolaee's other office. The nurse tells my parents that they have to stay in the waiting room because there is not enough space where I'm going to be examined.

It's a dark, chilly examination room, with most of the light projected from the machine's screen.

I sit on the lightly cushioned blue table and listen to the machine's hum. My heart rate is rising just from the uncertainty. Dr. Koolaee sees that I am nervous. "No need to worry," he says. "You've done this before. It's pretty much like a sonogram of your heart. What I'd like you to do is just lie back on the table."

Dr. Koolaee then applies a jellylike substance to my chest before affixing sticky electrode patches. "All you have to do is breathe normally and relax." He proceeds to roll a small rounded plastic device around the upper region of my rib cage. I hear a squishy thumping noise coming from the speakers. I'm assuming that this swishing noise is the sound of my heart pumping.

The echocardiogram takes about twenty minutes. Afterward, Dr. Koolaee tells me the verdict. "Your heart looks good. It shows a lot of improvement and progression since last time, which is really great. All the physical activity and fitness that you have been doing since you left the hospital has strengthened your heart."

"So that means I have your approval to go to Kona?" I ask.

"Yes, but as long as you promise not to overdo it. If you feel any signs of strain on your heart or lungs, any strain at all, stop right then and there. But from what I've seen here today, your heart looks good. I wish you the best of luck and I can't wait to hear how it goes."

I can't thank him enough.

He tells me he has only one request.

"Of course, what is it?"

"Could you bring me back a T-shirt from Hawaii?"

We walk out together to the waiting room. My parents appear nervous, but that instantly changes when they hear his prognosis: all systems go!

As soon as I get home, I call the Ironman's Peter Henning who says that the next step will be completing a half-Ironman triathlon. He suggests the Whirlpool Steelhead 70.3 Triathlon in Benton Harbor, Michigan, which takes place on August 5, 2007, and is little more than two weeks away.

Uh-oh. That doesn't give me much time to train. But I keep these doubts to myself. Peter then says that one of the Ironman gear sponsorship managers will call me on Monday.

When I hang up, I consider what I must now do. One hour a day on the stationary bike or treadmill is not going to be enough for a 70.3-mile race. I'm not worried about the open-water aspect of the triathlon because of my background in swimming. My main concern is the bike. As for the final segment of the race, the half-marathon run, well, I'm just going to have to give everything I have left to push through that third leg. But what does this really mean? I am in no shape to jog, let alone *run* more than a few miles. I wonder what 13.1 miles feel like anyway. Will my legs give out before the finish? I guess I won't know until I try.

So I start my training for a triathlon with an hourlong run on the treadmill, then an hour on the stationary bike, followed by thirty minutes of additional treadmill running. I'm totally beat afterward. My body is toast. If I'm spent from only two and a half hours of training, how in the world am I going to be able to complete a 70.3-mile triathlon? This is ridiculous. I am grossly illprepared and undertrained to do a triathlon, let alone a half-Ironman in two weeks. Yet what feverishly spurs me on is that vision of myself on life support in the ICU. If I had made it through that hell barely clinging to life, just how tough could a triathlon be in comparison? On the other hand, there's only so much I can ask of my body. Why push my luck?

The next day, I get a call from Andy Giancola, the Ironman sponsorship manager who will fix me up with a Cannondale triathlon bike.

All this is great news, but then the Boyles are hit hard by another setback. My Grandma Gladys is rushed to the hospital because of severe stomach pains. When I visit her in the hospital, many of my relatives are already there. As soon as I walk into her room, I smell her rose-scented perfume, which stops me right in my tracks. I move closer to her, sit down, and hold her frail hand.

She speaks first. "Brian, your Uncle Pat was telling me about your big race coming up." Her voice is weak.

"Yeah Grandma. But we can talk about all that later . . . how are you feeling?"

"I was just having a lot of pain in my stomach. More than usual I guess. I'll be okay," she says in her positive voice.

"I'd rather stay and be with you than go somewhere to do a triathlon."

"No, no. I'll be fine; don't worry about me. You have to do the race. I want you to tell me all about it when you get back."

I hold back tears and attempt to smile.

Over the next few days, I continue to train but I have Grandma constantly in my thoughts. I keep to a regular schedule of an hour on the stationary bike, an hour on the treadmill, and an hour in the backyard pool. I've also been receiving boxes of free gear from Ironman sponsors: PowerBars and PowerBar gels, TYR triathlon swimsuits and swim goggles, Cannondale bike clothing, Newton running shoes, Foster Grant sunglasses, and hydration belts and duffel bags from Nathan Sports.

I get a call from the local bike shop in Waldorf, Maryland, called the Bike Doctor. Chris Richardson says that my Cannondale CAAD8 bike is ready. My dad drives me to the shop. The bike has sleek racing features with aero bars jutting out from the handlebars like high-tech antlers. This exotic racing machine intimidates me.

Chris takes out a pair of bike shoes and demonstrates how to clip them into the pedals. It looks confusing.

I hop on the bike in the store, and Chris does some minor seat and handlebar adjustments for proper fit. He starts flicking through the gears while giving me a quick rundown of its features.

My dad helps me load the Cannondale in the back of his truck and we head over to the same high school track where we used to do our walking sessions after I was released from the hospital. The track's rubberized surface will be more forgiving should I take a tumble.

As he watches me get on the bike, I feel like a young kid riding a bike for the first time. The results are nearly the same. As soon as I push off, with my feet on top of the pedals, not inside them, I run into a fence.

I get back on the bike, kick off, and creep along. But I can only get one foot in the pedal and the bike halts. I fall. Oops.

The third time, I manage to get both feet into the pedals. I ride one lap but when I press the brakes and unclip my left foot, I lose my balance and slam into the fence. How am I ever going to ride fifty-six miles?

I'm back on the bike, riding along, flipping through the gears by clicking the metal shifting levers on the handlebars. I'm not exactly sure what I'm doing. It's a guessing game which gear I'm in. When I try riding crouched over with my forearms cradled in the aero bars, I feel like a praying mantis on wheels. The bike begins to wobble, so I lift my arms out of the aero bars and return to riding upright.

I end up riding for thirty minutes, which is all I will have time to do before the Michigan race. I hope it's an easy bike course without hills or sharp turns.

The next day, we drop off our bulldog puppy, Daisy, at the nearby kennel and then visit my grandma whose health is rapidly failing. I give her a hug. "Grandma, we're leaving tomorrow for the race," I tell her.

"I know you are," she says quietly, smiling.

"I'm going to finish the race for you, Grandma. I promise." I do my best to hold back tears.

My "Rushed" Two-Week* Training Diary for Steelhead Half-Ironman

MONDAY

Run

warm-up	easy jog 1 mile (15:00)
set	3 mile treadmill run (60:00)
cool down	easy jog 1 mile (15:00)

Weights

muscle	*exercise (2 sets of 15 reps)*
biceps	barbell curls
chest	bench press
triceps	upright rows

TUESDAY

Bike

warm-up	easy 1 mile (10:00)
set	stationary bike (60:00)
cool down	easy 1 mile (10:00)

Weights

muscle	*exercise (2 sets of 15 reps)*
upper and lower legs	squats
calves	calf raises
upper and lower legs	lunges

* I did the same workout for the second week, adding thirty minutes on the bike at the track.

WEDNESDAY

Swim (3200 yards)

warm-up	300 choice 300 free
drills	400 stroke technique 200 free catch up
set	12x25 free sprint intervals on 25 secs 10x50 free sprint intervals on 50 secs
kicking	4x200 free
set	2x100 free intervals 2 min
cool down	200 choice easy

Weights

muscle	exercise (2 sets of 15 reps)
biceps	barbell curls
chest	bench press
triceps	upright rows

THURSDAY

Run

warm-up	easy jog 1 mile (15:00)
set	3-mile treadmill run (60:00)
cool down	easy jog 1 mile (15:00)

Weights

muscle	exercise (2 sets of 15 reps)
upper and lower legs	squats
calves	calf raises
upper and lower legs	lunges

FRIDAY

Abs

crunches	3 x 25 reps
oblique crunches	3 x 25 reps
leg raises	3 x 25 reps

Bike

warm-up	easy 1 mile (10:00)
set	stationary bike (60:00)
cool down	easy 1 mile (10:00)

Weights

muscle	*exercise (2 sets of 15 reps)*
biceps	barbell curls
chest	bench press
triceps	upright rows

SATURDAY

Swim (4100 yards)

warm-up	300 stroke 300 free
drills	10x50 free, rest: 25 secs 25 slow—25 fast
set	12x25 sprint free intervals.50 secs 10x50 sprint free intervals. 95 secs
pulling	8x100, rest: 25 secomds
set	400 IM, rest 60 secs 4x100 free, rest: 15 secs 8x50 free sprint, rest: 30 secs
cool down	200 choice easy

Weights

muscle	exercise (2 sets of 15 reps)
upper and lower legs	squats
calves	calf raises
upper and lower legs	lunges

SUNDAY
Rest

WE GET UP EARLY AT THREE O'CLOCK TO CATCH AN EARLY FLIGHT TO Kalamazoo, Michigan. Airport security at Reagan National rifles through my black TYR duffel bag and removes all my PowerBar gels. Inexplicably, they are on the forbidden list of TSA carry-on items.

After we land, we check into the hotel in Benton Harbor, which is on the eastern shore of Lake Michigan and also the administrative home of the triathlon's title sponsor, Whirlpool Corporation. In the hotel room, my dad and I try to reassemble the Cannondale bike but we're hopelessly confused. The following morning, we drop it off at a local bike shop, then register for the triathlon at race headquarters in Jean Klock Park.

I definitely feel out of place among all these tanned, super-fit triathletes. They appear confident, which is one attribute I desperately lack. I wish I wasn't so bulked up from weightlifting. I have to ask several people where I must go and what I need to do for the race.

I decide it would be a good idea to practice swimming in my Blue Seventy wetsuit for the first time. Squeezing my 220 pounds inside a skintight wetsuit requires my parents' assistance. It feels like the wetsuit will burst at any moment, but once I'm in the water, the neoprene wetsuit acts like a second layer of skin; it's insulating and adds buoyancy. There are other triathletes in the water and I follow their lead, loosening up with twenty minutes of freestyle. I swim to the beach to practice running in and out of the water, priming my legs because I'm used to just jumping off a starting block in swim meets. Here, it's a running beach start.

Once we get back to the hotel, I lay out everything for the next morning: wetsuit, race suit, ankle timing transponder, goggles and swim cap, bike helmet, bib number on race belt, bike shoes and socks, running shoes, sunglasses, visor, another pair of socks, watch, PowerBar gels, and sunscreen. For dinner, we drive to a local Italian restaurant for take-out spaghetti. I'm not really sure what triathletes eat before a race, but I always ate spaghetti on the eve of big swim meets.

It's still dark when we arrive at the race site. Dense knots of triathletes mill about, getting their bodies inked with race numbers, setting up their individual transition areas, fiddling with their bikes, pumping air in tires. Huge bright lights make the scene look like a movie set.

I go over to my bike in the transition area. It rained earlier, so I take a towel out of my bag to dry the handlebars and seat. I then place my bike and running shoes on the ground next to my bike, take out my helmet and place it on my bike's handlebars, and spray some sunscreen on my arms, shoulders, and face. I position my sunglasses and visor next to my shoes. I can't help but wonder if I am forgetting something.

I walk over to the beach starting area. Oasis's "Wonderwall" is blasting from concert speakers. Armies of wetsuit-clad triathletes are massing everywhere, numbering at least two thousand. I'm 99.9 percent sure that they all have more than several weeks of training under their belts.

Race officials align everyone on the beach in separate age-group-determined waves, denoted by the color of our swim caps. I'm in the eighteen-to-twenty-four category and wearing silver. We will be the third group to enter the lake for the 1.2-mile swim.

Beep! The sound of the air horn goes off and I stare in awe as the first triathlete group—the pros—make a fast dash across the sand toward the water, pushing and aggressively shoving one another.

Beep! The next group, all wearing red caps, go in at a much more relaxed pace. I think they are the women in my age group, but I'm not quite sure because I can only see a blur of people running toward the water.

Beep! It's my group's turn to make the rough voyage out. There is pushing, shoving, bumping, colliding. As soon as I hit the cold water, I find a surge of adrenaline and start cranking. I look for a safe patch of water where I won't get bludgeoned and bashed by other swimmers. The water is churning as if by a frenzied pack of starving piranhas.

Instead of all-out speed like in a fifty-yard freestyle race, I focus more on gliding with each stroke since the wetsuit's increased buoyancy allows me to ride higher in the water. This is unlike pool swimming. After about a minute, a hand strikes my cheekbone, which pops off my goggle's right side, letting cold water dribble in. "Dammit!" I yell underwater, though only bubbles explode from my mouth. Enraged, I keep swimming with limited vision, catch up to that guy, and swim past him while giving him a forceful nudge. I then feel a hard kick by my hip and I realize there are people swimming all around me. Smack! Another blow—to my neck and shoulders. I'm being flutter-kicked repeatedly. I quickly do a few strokes with my head poking out of the water while fixing the goggles. I finally find water where I'm not getting kicked or hit. I regain my rhythm. One stroke, two strokes, three strokes, breathe, repeat.

Some swimmers are drafting right behind other people's feet. Is this to go faster? It looks difficult to swim that way, especially when all those bubbles explode in your face. What if the person you're swimming behind is going off course—then what?

Every time I lift my head to breathe, I'm greeted by the sun's orange disc hanging low in the sky. Wow, what a sight. I've never experienced that kind of view while swimming laps.

I pass an orange buoy. A swimmer on my left comes too close for comfort as we round the buoy and our arms keep colliding. What's his problem? I elongate my stroke and edge past him.

I sneak a glimpse of my watch—27:12. Then, *bam*! My mind takes an unexpected detour and visions of being back in the hospital intrude. Three years ago, I was on my deathbed, and now I'm swimming in Lake Michigan. If somebody came into my hospital room back then and said, "Someday you will be competing in a half-Ironman triathlon," I would have considered that a cruel, sadistic joke.

"Just keep swimming; just keep swimming," I repeat over and over in my mind. Where is that line from? Oh, that's right! It's from the *Finding Nemo* soundtrack. Then it's onto the drum solo in Led Zeppelin's "Moby Dick."

My goggles begin to fog. Luckily, it happens close to the beach. When my right hand rotates around and dives down in the water, it picks up a handful of sand. Land! Hallelujah!

I stand, but my legs are Jell-O. I fall back in the water and do a belly flop. I get back on my knees, disoriented, and crawl through the shallow water until I stumble back on my feet. I jog up the beach across red carpet mats. I feel so dizzy that any second I could throw up. Too late. I stop, bend over, and dry heave, but fortunately nothing comes up.

"Hey Brian! Over here!" The voice comes from my right. I look over and see my mom and dad. I wave to them and head over to the bike corral.

As I fumble taking off my wetsuit, I hear someone else shout, "Hey Brian, how are you doing?" I look around and see a guy standing near the bike rack. He's wearing a red Ironman triathlon cap, dark sunglasses, a navy blue polo shirt with the Ironman logo, and a pair of dark gray khakis. "It's me, Peter Henning." He walks up and shakes my hand.

"Mr. Henning! It's great to finally meet you." We begin having a casual conversation as if the triathlon isn't taking place. I slip on my bike shorts, jersey, socks, shoes, helmet, and sunglasses. "It's a nice day for a bike ride," I add, while munching down a PowerBar. Meanwhile, a long ribbon of triathletes continues to funnel through the bike corral; they tear off their wetsuits, change into bike gear, and jog off with their bikes toward the transition area exit. I realize I should get going.

"Aren't you forgetting something?" says Peter, handing me my race bib number. I stop to wrap it around my race belt and attach it in the front. I wheel my bike out on the asphalt road, but as I lift my right leg over the top tube and seat, I clumsily high-kick the Gatorade bottle off the back of my seat. Because I'm not used to running and walking in bike shoes, I leave the bottle on the ground. I have another.

It's a losing battle to get both feet clipped into the pedals. Left foot is in, but I'm a zigzagging danger to other competitors. I'm teetering like a drunk, nearly plowing into a group of three riders. "Hey watch it!" one yells in disgust. I lower my head in shame and furiously hurry to click my right foot into the other pedal. I'm barely moving until I finally hear a click. Now I'm in business. In the meantime, about fifty triathletes have zoomed right by.

As I flick through the cog selections to find the correct gear, I sit upright like I'm riding a beach cruiser. The other riders are bent over their aero bars, slicing through the air. I can't chance riding that way—I'd be a safety hazard to the triathletes who are flying by in a kaleidoscopic blur.

The bike course travels through a series of small neighborhoods, back roads, and small streets where police monitor the traffic at each stoplight. On slight curves, I slow down. On straightaways, I pedal faster and reach a regular rhythm. This section of southwest Michigan is known as the fruit belt and includes blueberry, strawberry, and raspberry farms, as well as vineyards and orchards.

Within an hour, I must be passed by over two hundred riders, and the number increases every minute. The only people I've passed are several racers fixing flats by the side of the road. What would happen if I got a flat? It would be disastrous.

I keep both hands glued to the handlebars since my bike-handling ability remains shaky. The slightest movement in steering throws me off-balance.

I pass an aid station where volunteers hand out bottles of water and Gatorade, but as badly as I want to reach out and grab one, I'm afraid of running into people. I smile politely and keep going.

But it's getting hot, over eighty degrees. My black bike shorts have turned white from all the sodium that I've lost from sweating. A Gatorade bottle sits in the downtube cage, but I'm too nervous to reach down for it. So my thirst mounts, reminding me of when I was in Intensive Care and forced to spend endless hours dreaming about having a sip of water from the nearby sink. It's happening again—a drink just out of reach.

I'm also famished. I have been riding for over two hours. A PowerBar and several PowerBar gels are nestled in a small black bag attached to the handlebars. Food is tantalizing close, but there's absolutely no way I'm going to ride one-handed.

Drained of energy and strength, I'm getting progressively more dizzy and nauseous. I'm not sweating anymore, but feel cold and clammy, a sure sign of approaching dehydration and heat exhaustion. My legs feel like rotating anvils.

At the next aid station, I'm determined to get something to drink. I slow to a crawl, release my right hand from the handlebars, and timidly raise it a few inches. In a leap of faith, I launch my arm and grab a water bottle from a volunteer's outstretched hand. I hold the bottle close to my chest before chugging down its entire contents in three continuous gulps.

Several more miles and at long last, there's a most welcome sight for this boy from Welcome, Maryland. Just ahead is the bike-to-run transition area. I made it! Fifty-six miles!

Thousands of spectators line the park. I notice Peter Henning and an NBC camera guy filming. Now that I'm on camera, I pretend that I'm Mr. Cool rather than fatigued and hurting. As I brake to a halt and attempt to plant both feet on the ground, I slip and fall. Peter rushes over to see if I'm okay. I tell him that I'm good to go as I start hopping away, scraped and bruised, with my bike rolling alongside me.

I place my bike into the rack, then sit down for a quick meal of two PowerBars and PowerBar gels. I remove my bike helmet and lace up my running shoes. Peter walks over. He says that I finished the bike ride in almost three-and-a-half hours—an average speed of sixteen miles per hour—as he helps me stand because my legs are locked tight. I feel like the Tin Man in the *Wizard of Oz* before he gets his can of oil.

I jog out of the transition area. I see my parents and throw them a wave and smile. My jogging is more like bouncing from one foot to the other because my knees won't extend much. My legs have just finished spinning in tiny circles all morning. Of course, they want to remain uncooperative.

Several other triathletes are also lumbering at my pace. They appear to be in their forties and fifties. We're back-of-the-packers. It's been a long while since I have seen any guys in my age group.

At mile two, a steep hill wants to break my resolve. Jogging is replaced by walking. When I reach the top, I hum the theme song to *Rocky*.

The run course follows the St. Joseph River. Each mile takes me about twenty minutes. By letting gravity do the work, my body falls forward and then catches itself before it hits the road. That's how I cover ground with numb legs.

Exhausted and aching all over, I find myself replaying painful periods from the coma and recovery. As I grind past the fourth, fifth, and sixth mile markers, I think about all the people who have helped me along the way—my parents, doctors, nurses, rehab therapists, friends.

I hear my dad's voice from the hospital in a continuous loop: "We all know how much you're hurting right now; we know you're in pain, but you have to keep fighting. Don't give up."

Mile nine. I stop at the aid station and splash three cups of water on my face, head, and under my shirt. I grab a handful of ice-cold sponges and stuff them under my jersey. I down two cups of Gatorade, take a bite of banana, suck an orange slice, and squeeze a PowerBar gel into my mouth. It must be ninety degrees. The sun is cooking my skin lobster-red.

Mile ten. My dad's voice from Intensive Care returns. "Come on now, you can beat this; we know you can. We have been here by your side every day."

I've stopped all pretense of jogging. Instead, I scrape my feet along the hot asphalt pavement.

Mile eleven. I'm a walking, stumbling corpse. My dad's voice again from the hospital: "You can do it son."

Mile twelve. One more mile to go before the torment ends.

The finish line is near. The announcer screams out each person's name as he or she crosses the line. Buoyed by the spectators cheering, my death walk turns into a stiff-legged jog.

Mile 13.1. I cross the finish line. The announcer booms, "Brian Boyle from Welcome, Maryland, has crossed the line at seven hours and thirteen minutes."

Peter Henning rushes over and congratulates me. The NBC camera zeroes in on me. My parents emerge from behind the spectator fence and embrace me. My mom is sobbing; these are tears of joy, not sadness. My dad proudly pats me on the back. A small team of race volunteers wrap a towel around my shoulders, unravel the timing chip from my shoelaces, and place a shiny finisher's medal around my neck. I'm wobbly. I need to sit down somewhere. But before I depart, Peter asks, "Because the Hawaii Ironman is *twice* the distance of the Steelhead 70.3, do you think you could go back out there and do the race all over again?"

I respond with a huge grin. "Twice as far? Yes, of course. Just give me another two weeks to train." We all start laughing. My mother's tear-stained cheeks are glistening in the bright sunshine.

Kona, here I come.

CHAPTER 30

FROM COMA TO KONA

I'VE PAID DEARLY FOR THE STEELHEAD HALF-IRONMAN BY PUSHING MY body almost to the breaking point. For several days afterward, my legs are wooden and sore, my lower back hurts, my neck is out of whack, my feet look like raw hamburger, and several toenails go black before falling off. I'm back to shuffling around like I did for months following my release from the hospital. Fortunately, I don't need a cane or wheelchair. By week's end, my body's fully recovered.

My grandma's health, however, refuses to rebound. Doctors have determined she has pancreatic cancer, and it's terminal. She has been moved from the hospital to hospice care at her home in Oxon Hill. My parents and I visit her right after returning from Michigan. I bring my Steelhead finisher's medal to show her.

She looks much thinner and the cancer is spreading quickly. She smiles when she sees us. Her bedroom is filled with all my aunts, uncles, and cousins. I place my finisher's medal in her right hand. When she feels the cool metal in her palm, she feebly wraps her fingers around it, but she's too weak to speak. Two days later, she is gone.

Around this time, Henning calls, informing me that I've been granted one of the coveted NBC media slots for the 2007 Ironman World Championship in Kona, Hawaii on October 13. That's the good news. The bad news is that the race is only forty-five days away. It will be a race simply to see if I can make it to the starting line in one piece. At my grandma's funeral service, I lean over her pearl-white casket and tell her that she will be with me in spirit on the Big Island.

The Ironman folks place me in direct contact with their official coaches from LifeSport because they want to ensure that I'm adequately prepared for Kona. I have less than two months to whip my body into shape. This will be like cramming for a final exam, except this test takes all day to complete. LifeSport's founder and head coach, Lance Watson, trained Canadian Olympic triathlon gold-medal winner Simon Whitfield to his victory in Sydney and now trains Ironman champion Lisa Bentley. I just want to survive Hawaii. By the time the pros finish and are getting their massages, I'll just be starting the marathon. I'm not out for glory, just to finish.

I do some rough math. Of the 1,870 Steelhead triathletes who started that half-Ironman race, I finished in 1,707th place, or the bottom 15 percent. I was far from last. My time was 7:13:20. So double that and add an extra hour for Hawaii's heat, wind, and exhaustion, and I hope to complete the Ironman in just over fifteen hours. The race starts with a 2.4-mile swim in the choppy Pacific Ocean. Rush out of the water, dash through a shower to rinse off the salt, change clothes, jump onto a bicycle, and pedal for 112 miles through a lava desert. To finish, you'll need to run a hot, windy 26.2 miles. The fastest pros will complete the race in a little over eight hours, and the last person will hopefully finish by midnight, or in seventeen hours—the official cut-off time.

Each day, I receive an email from LifeSport with a list of suggested workouts. Some routines consist of a forty-five-minute run followed by a weight-training session in my home gym. The next day might be an hour swim in the backyard pool followed by a long bike ride at the local high school track. I'm still too green to risk riding a bike on the local country roads. My parents emphatically agree; they want to keep me far away from traffic.

So around and around the high school track I go on my Cannondale CAAD8, lap after lap, sometimes for two or three hours. This seems like sheer lunacy, but I have no other option. Some of the runners look at me like I'm crazy, but they eventually get accustomed to my two-wheel presence. The good news is that I'm gradually acquiring the skill and confidence to ride tucked into the aero position, clicking gears up and down with a better understanding of their intended purpose. I've also improved my balance so I can consistently ride in a straight line. The track's white lane lanes are a great help. Memories of Steelhead when I almost ran into people in the bike transition zone haunt me.

LifeSport also recommends that I do longer weekend workouts called "bricks," which involve cycling five hours followed by a thirty-minute run. There is no way I can ride for five hours around the quarter-mile track, so I expand the bike course to include the school parking lot and private road, which is maybe a half-mile long. On weekends, this works well because school isn't in session and I have the road all to myself. My dad often rides alongside me on his mountain bike.

To train for Steelhead, I only ran indoors on the treadmill. That has to change for Hawaii. But once again, my parents have a justifiable concern about my not running on the road with traffic. So I do all my marathon preparations for Kona in my neighborhood where there are only ten houses. The road is one mile long. It takes eleven minutes to run its length. My neighbors often wave to me as I run back and forth. There's virtually no traffic, maybe a car every hour.

It's an awkward transition to go from the treadmill to the road because I'm used to the treadmill's bounce and cushion, so my joints are a little sore at first. Running up to eight lengths along the same road is mind-numbing, so I usually bring along my iPod, which I keep attached to an armband around my bicep. I usually start my training with Alice in Chains's "Rooster" or AC/DC's "For Those About to Rock." By the workout's end, I'm listening to Judas Priest's "Delivering the Goods" or Pantera's "Revolution is My Name."

I relied on my swimming background at Steelhead. But I have to increase my mileage for Hawaii. Since my swim time for 1.2 miles in Steelhead was around thirty-nine minutes, I estimate that my time in Kona will be a little more than double that—around one hour and twenty minutes. When I trained in high school and college, I'd swim continuously for up to twenty minutes, but now I'm swimming for over an hour in the pool. I often go to the high school pool where Sam is the lifeguard. For some workouts, I only use my arms, swimming with a pull buoy held between my legs. The pull buoy is a light floatation device to keep the body upright so the body won't sink when the legs aren't kicking. With open-water swimming, you want your arms doing most of the work in order to keep your legs fresh for the bike and run. With the pull buoy, I swim anywhere from four laps to fifty laps, then alternate with regular front-crawl swimming between twenty and a hundred laps.

After my bruising experience in Lake Michigan, when I was knocked about by other swimmers like laundry in a washing machine, I've prepared myself for the swim start's free-for-all. I have my younger cousins smack me with foam bats and repeatedly jump on me from the sides of our backyard pool as I swim laps.

Besides swimming, biking, and running, I'm also improving my lung strength by doing various exercises in the backyard pool. Since our pool is eight feet in the deep end and four feet in the shallow end, I run from the shallow end to the deep end underwater while holding a twenty-five-pound weight against my chest that keeps me submerged. My inspiration for this type of workout came from watching surfing films when I was growing up. These movies showed Hawaiian surfers training to improve their lung strength and endurance by going out to a spot in the ocean that's about ten feet deep, grabbing a large rock and running along the sandy bottom for as long as they could to strengthen their lungs. This was good preparation for when a surfer got knocked off his board and pinned underwater by crashing waves.

As the autumn days become shorter and the leaves begin to change colors, my body is also undergoing an alteration from all the triathlon training. I have lost about twenty pounds. I can run about a ten-minute mile. I'm a lot more efficient on the bike. My only hope is that these improvements will get me through the Ironman in under seventeen hours. Still, was six weeks sufficient time to train? Was I setting myself up for failure and a crushing, collosal disappointment? Why didn't I refuse Peter Henning when he offered me the Ironman slot? I could have thanked him and told him I wasn't ready. I could have told him maybe in a year or so, but not now. Where was that inner voice saying, "slow down, Brian"? My only plausible answer is that I'm supposed to be dead, like I've been living on borrowed time ever since the accident. This means that when an opportunity like the Ironman presents itself, I must accept the challenge without reservation or delay. Rejection or anything else only serves to reinforce the painful memories from the past, a past from which I can't help but flee like a fugitive.

A Sample Week of My Ironman Training

MONDAY

Abs

crunches	3 x 25
oblique crunches	3 x 25
leg raises	3 x 25

Run

warm-up	easy jog 1 mile (10:00)
set	3-mile run
cool down	easy jog 1 mile (10:00)

Weights

muscle	exercise (4 sets of 8 reps)
biceps	barbell curls
chest	bench press
triceps	upright rows

TUESDAY

Bike

warm-up	easy 1 mile (10:00)
set	1 hour bike
cool down	easy 1 mile (10:00)

Weights

muscle	*exercise (4 sets of 8 reps)*
upper and lower legs	squats
calves	calf raises
upper and lower legs	lunges

WEDNESDAY

Abs

crunches	3 x 25
oblique crunches	3 x 25
leg raises	3 x 25

Swim (5,100 yards)

warm-up	500 choice 500 free
drills	600 stroke 400 free catch up
set	12x25 free sprint intervals. 50 secs 20x50 free sprint intervals. 75 secs
kicking	4x300 free rest:1 min
set	4x100 free fast intervals 4 min
cool down	200 choice easy

Weights

muscle	exercise (4 sets of 8 reps)
biceps	barbell curls
chest	bench press
triceps	upright rows

THURSDAY

Run

warm-up	easy jog 1 mile (10:00)
set	6-mile run
cool down	easy jog 1 mile (10:00)

Weights

muscle	exercise (4 sets of 8 reps)
upper and lower legs	squats
calves	calf raises
upper and lower legs	lunges

FRIDAY

Rest

SATURDAY

Abs

crunches	3 x 25
oblique crunches	3 x 25
leg raises	3 x 25

Bike

warm-up	easy 1 mile (10:00)
set	4 hour bike
cool down	easy 1 mile (10:00)

Run

set	3-mile run

SUNDAY

Swim (5800 yards)

warm-up	500 stroke 500 free
drills	16x50 free rest 25 secs 25 slow - 25 fast
set	12x25 free sprint int. 50 secs 10x50 free sprint int. 95 secs
pulling	12x100 free rest 25 secs
set	400 IM rest 60 secs 8x100 free rest 20 secs 12x50 free sprint rest 30 secs
cool down	200 choice easy

Weights

muscle	*exercise (4 sets of 8 reps)*
upper and lower legs	squats
calves	calf raises
upper and lower legs	lunges

OCTOBER 6, 2007. I ARRIVE WITH MY PARENTS IN KONA, HAWAII, ONE week before race day. It's three in the morning when the plane lands at Keahole Airport. My jet-lagged sleepy brain is locked within a state of disbelief when my feet touch the tarmac. In the dark, humid night I feel confusion, even intense disorientation. Everything seems unreal. Just being here feels like a dream. Just over three years ago, I was waking up from a coma. Everything was puzzling and strange in the hospital room. Nothing made sense. I didn't know where I was, how I got there, why I couldn't move any of my limbs. But there's a big difference between coma and Kona. I didn't ask to land in a coma. A speeding dump truck made that happen. But I *want* to be in Kona. I've worked hard at it, fighting against steep odds. I have had tremendous help along the way, from the doctors and nurses when I was smashed and crushed, to the generous assistance from the Ironman organization. While I'm not an elite age-grouper who qualified for Hawaii, I feel as fortunate and as lucky as any of the other 150 lottery winners who snagged an entry slot.

I am grateful that my parents are with me in Kona. They have made this long journey with me at all times, from Room 19 in Intensive Care at Prince George's Hospital to our adjacent rooms at the King Kamehameha Hotel, which is also race headquarters for the Hawaii Ironman Triathlon World Championship.

I fall asleep right after checking into my room. The next thing I know, I'm having a dream. I'm alone on a sailboat in waters off the Hawaiian coast. The boat is fairly beaten up. The mainsail and jib aren't out because there isn't much wind. The anchor line is taut as it enters the clear blue water. Various pieces of nautical equipment are on board—old buoys and a sun-bleached life raft. I notice small, white-painted lava rocks scattered across the scuffed oak floor. Suddenly, I get this powerful urge for a drink of water, but there's nothing to drink on the boat. So I decide to swim to shore and find fresh water. I prop my hands over the carved oak hull, and am ready to jump overboard when I see an engraving in the wood next to my left foot. It says July 6. I lose my balance and fall backward into the ocean.

The dream ends. I look over to the alarm clock on the nightstand. It's almost six in the morning—time to wake up. In several hours, I will begin the first session of a four-day Ironman training camp.

I meet my fellow LifeSport campers in the lobby of the hotel. Our instructors are LifeSport's Lance Watson, Paul Regensburg, and Alister Russell, who will help newcomers like myself become familiar with the race course. There are fifteen triathletes in the camp, men and women, old and young, and judging from their accents, from all over the world—United States, Canada, Australia, and New Zealand. The skill levels are broad, ranging from lottery-slot recipients to elite age-groupers and even a few professionals. I'm both the youngest and the least conditioned triathlete. I'm the baby of the group.

Our first training session takes place at the Natural Energy Lab of Hawaii, which conducts cutting-edge research in small-scale ocean thermal energy. The 870-acre complex spreads out from the seashore to the Queen Ka'ahumanu ("Queen K") Highway, which is the main road for the bike and run course. The three-mile asphalt spur to the Energy Lab—coming at the sixteen-mile mark in the marathon—is where many Ironman champions have been born.

Several campers all tell me the same thing: This place should be called anything but the Energy Lab because that is the last thing you have left in your tank during the marathon. They're probably right.

The flat road that descends to the sea is scorched and charred earth, the remnants of a volcanic eruption that happened two hundred years ago. We park the van. Campers pile out and immediately start running. Some move blazingly fast, galloping along at a six-minutes-per-mile pace. They all have quick leg turnover, land on their mid-foot, and run with nice long strides. My form is pitiful: slow leg turnover, short strides, and I periodically land on my heels.

I begin with a light jog in this South Sea sauna whose heat sucks away my breath. I return to the van after twenty minutes, overheated and drained. The other campers are busy chatting, their arms and legs glistening with sweat and liquefied sunscreen. They don't even look tired.

"How was the run?" asks a super-fast Aussie named Brad. "It's hot, mate. It's burnin' up out here."

"Yeah, it's pretty warm," I reply, with sweat dripping down my face.

When we get back to the hotel, we take a short break. I use the time to walk around the small town of Kona. Triathletes are everywhere, walking around with their bikes, helmets on or slung over their shoulders, carrying duffel bags with bike pump handles hanging out of them, and wearing running or bike jerseys. They are speaking German, French, Japanese, English, and Spanish. One young couple wear T-shirts that proclaim Tri or Die with a skull and crossbones printed in black.

I poke my head into the souvenir shops. I see triathletes chatting at small tables in outdoor cafes with their shiny bikes propped next to their chairs. Many of the guys aren't wearing shirts, so you can see their heart-rate monitor tan lines—a band of white stretching across their muscular chests. The girls are wearing sporty tank tops. They all have lean, flat abs. I feel like a foreigner, just another stocky tourist, among these chiseled bodies. I'm not in Maryland anymore.

Tropical trees and bright flowers line both sides of the main seaside road, Alii Drive. In less than a week, I will be running along this road that hugs the coast. For now, I allow my senses to be swept away by the aroma of seafood and coffee. People of all ethnicities smile at me as I walk the streets of Kona, and I return their friendly gestures. For the first time since waking up from the accident, I'm at absolute peace with myself.

I veer off the sidewalk and shopping area and find a perch on a concrete seawall. Kailua Bay is calm and looks like a sheet of rolling glass from the way the sun strikes the surface. I watch two swimmers stroking along in a good strong rhythm. Sitting alone, I become hypnotized by these faraway swimmers, their arms regularly rising over the blue water. The longer I stare at them, the more thankful I feel.

ON THE CAMP'S SECOND DAY OF TRAINING, WE MEET AT THE KONA PIER in the afternoon to learn more about the swim course. The large bright orange buoys are already in place. I can't even see the last buoy. I'm told it's yellow.

"Hey Brad, can you see the last buoy out there?" I ask, as he adjusts his swim goggles.

"Nah, mate. I was just getting ready to ask you the same thing," he says, and we both let out a nervous chuckle.

As I wade into Kailua Bay, I find the water cool and refreshing. I'm used to swimming in a pool, so the first thing that I notice is that I'm more buoyant in the salt water. I can rotate my arms at a regular freestyle pace but it seems easier.

There are several dozen triathletes swimming, keeping close to the buoys. I see tropical fish when I look down. It's a spectacular view—one

I never had swimming in pools, where the only feature is a single black line. There are small rolling waves. I can't imagine what things would be like if the waves were bigger.

Lance, Alister, and Paul accompany us in one-person kayaks. Lance says we should try drafting. We are paired into partners and instructed to swim for about fifty yards. Brad and I team up.

I have to race to keep up with Brad's feet, trying to catch the exploding bubbles with my cupped hands. Occasionally, I touch his toes, and he then increases his pace. This is a great workout for speed and technique. I switch places with Brad and now I'm the one being chased. There's a noticeable difference when I have to cut through the water by myself. Drafting works. Brad and I alternate back and forth all the way back to the shore.

As I towel off my hair, I run into professional triathlete Joanna Zeiger, with whom I've been corresponding via email. She and her husband Mark Shenk are good friends with one of my St. Mary's classmates, Montse Ferrer. Joanna turned pro in 1998 after being voted 1997 amateur triathlete of the year, excelling in all three distances of triathlon: Olympic, half-Ironman, and Ironman. In 2000, she won triathlete of the year honors for her fourth-place finish in the Olympics in Sydney and her fifth-place finish six weeks later in Kona for the Ironman World Championship. In 2005, she won her first Ironman in Brazil and then won Ironman Coeur d'Alene in 2006. And now in 2007, she is back in Kona.

She is pleased to see me. Wishing that I do well, she runs down a list of race tips, including what to have for breakfast on race day, how to take salt pills to avoid leg cramps during the bike and run, how often I should eat and drink, and how to maintain proper foot cadence during the marathon.

THOUGH IT'S ONLY MY SECOND DAY IN KONA, IRONMAN'S DIRECTOR OF communications, Blair LaHaye, has asked me to attend a special Ironman "Inspirational Triathletes" press conference. A large room off the hotel lobby is set up for the conference. I take a seat at the front table with three other triathletes. Blair introduces us to the gathered reporters and news media with brief biographies.

The first person Blair introduces is Scott Johnson, an accomplished Ironman triathlete from North Carolina in his mid-thirties who has cystic fibrosis and is also a double lung transplant recipient. He recently completed the Ironman Florida in Panama City Beach in a time of 15:00:50. This is his first time in Kona.

The next athlete is Scott Rigsby, who is also in his mid-thirties and is from Georgia. He's an experienced triathlete who will be the first below-the-knee double leg amputee to do Ironman with prosthetics. He lost both legs in an auto accident when he was eighteen years old.

Blair then introduces the older man to my right, Charlie Plaskon, who is a sixty-five-year-old grandfather and former schoolteacher who was diagnosed with a form of macular dystrophy called Stargardt's disease when he was six years old. After retiring from the classroom, the Florida resident took up running and triathlon. Since 2003, he has completed numerous marathons and triathlons. Because he's legally blind, he must swim and run with his guide, Matt Miller. When it's time to bike, Charlie pedals on the tandem's rear.

Sitting at the podium and listening to these three men talk about their experiences and how they have overcome physical limitations makes me feel proud to do this race with them. We share an intense connection, a bond of determination and willpower. Each one of us was forced to go far beyond what most thought we were capable of.

Then Blair introduces me: "Just three years ago, Brian Boyle was involved in a serious car accident. . . . "

I feel butterflies fluttering in my stomach. Over a hundred journalists are here. Cameras are pointed at me, with flashes going off every few seconds. I have no experience being in the media spotlight like this. I'm terrified. Blair hands me the microphone.

I nervously begin: "On July 6, 2004, one month after graduating from high school, I was driving home from swim practice when I was involved in a near-fatal car accident with a dump truck. My heart was knocked across my chest, my lungs collapsed, and my pelvis and left clavicle were shattered. Pretty much every organ in my body was damaged. I lost 60 percent of my blood and was medevacked out of the intersection and flown to a local shock trauma unit. I underwent fourteen operations during a two-month ordeal during which I was in a chemically induced coma and on life support.

"My three goals after graduating high school were to go to college, swim on the team, and to one day do an Ironman triathlon. But after the accident, these dreams were gone. I've miraculously accomplished two of these goals with a lot of help and support from my parents, family, and friends, and now I'm trying to realize my third."

I conclude by saying, "It's an absolute honor to be here in Kona competing with the world's best triathletes and to be given the chance to live a dream. Scott Johnson, Scott Rigsby, and Charlie Plaskon, I wish you all the best for this weekend's race and that we will all get to the finish line together. I would like to thank the Ironman for allowing me to be here, and I would like to thank my parents for always believing in me. It's an absolute honor and privilege to be here. Thank you all for making it possible."

After a round of applause for all four of us, there is no time for me to stay around and answer reporters' questions because I have an interview scheduled with Ron Staton of the Associated Press.

Right from the start, Ron puts me at ease with his gentle conversational manner. He asks me questions about training, the hospital, rehab, the half-Ironman Steelhead race in Michigan, and my plans after I finish the Ironman. And then he asks, "What if you *don't* finish?" This last question stumps me. I tell him that I will have to get back to him on that.

After our interview, I can't help but mull over this last question. *What if I don't finish?* I have been so absorbed with getting to Kona, I never really thought about not finishing. I can't now let doubts creep into my mind, because they could affect me psychologically on race day. No, I'm going to finish this race. But my main legitimate concern is avoiding a bike crash.

The next morning, I find a copy of the *West Hawaii Today* newspaper by my door. On the front page of the sports section is Ron's article, "From Alpha to Ambitious," along with several photos of me. I hurry to show the profile to my parents. We are thrilled.

I then check my email to find around fifty emails from friends, relatives, and school acquaintances who have read the article. My story also appears on ESPN.com, SportsIllustrated.com, and CNN.com. When I listen to my voicemail, I have seventeen messages from newspapers, radio stations, and local news stations in Baltimore and Washington, D.C. They all want to interview me.

ON THE THIRD DAY OF THE LIFESPORT CAMP, LANCE BIKES ALONGSIDE me on the Queen K Highway, giving me pointers on how to better shift gears, how to get my body more streamlined, and how to efficiently switch water bottles when one gets empty. Even though the race is still several days away, the road is jammed with cyclists in training. Every few minutes, I hear somebody behind me shout "left" in English or the equivalent in their native language, and I try to scoot over and let the rider pass.

CANNONDALE'S MARKETING MANAGER, BILL RUDELL, IS IN KONA AND phones me at the hotel to meet him at the local bike shop called Bike Works. When I arrive, the place is swarming with triathletes. Most of them are in cycling jerseys, walking awkwardly in their bike shoes, and still wearing their helmets. Everyone has a fancy triathlon bike, and is hoping to get minor prerace mechanical adjustments.

"Hey, Brian, is that you? Over here buddy." I hear a cheerful voice coming from the side of the bike shop. A guy in a gray baseball cap, a black Cannondale T-shirt, tan cargo shorts, and a pair of flip-flops approaches. It's Rudell.

"It's great to finally meet you!" I say enthusiastically, as I shake his hand and introduce him to my parents.

He leads us to the side of the building where Cannondale mechanics have set up a workstation. He points to a high-tech, extremely lightweight triathlon bike that's glimmering in the bright sunlight. "It's all yours, Brian, top of the line, our Slice," he says. "It's our most advanced and aerodynamic bike. Use it instead of the CAAD8."

I'm speechless.

"This bike won't even be available to the public for another two months," Bill says.

I pick it up. It's featherlight.

For the next forty-five minutes, Bill and his crew make minor adjustments with the bike setup while I sit in the saddle. They want me to be as comfortable as possible. We then load the bike into my parents' SUV rental to road test the Slice on the Queen K Highway.

I carefully lift my leg over the bike seat with that same apprehension as when I first climbed onto the CAAD8 in early August. I clip my left foot into the pedal and push off with my right, quickly picking up speed. The steering is extra tight and shaky. I start clicking through the gear levers, which are located at the ends of the aero bars extending out front of the regular handlebars. I try to crouch in the aero position, but it feels too forced and unfamiliar, so I remain upright.

I bike for about fifteen minutes while my parents trail behind in the SUV. Thankfully, the traffic is light. I finally get the confidence to lean forward into the aero position and I wrap my fingers around the gear levers.

Then *whoosh*! A big tractor-trailer passes on my left, and the windy wake causes me to wobble all over the shoulder. It's lucky I don't crash. I slam on the brakes and hop off the bike. I'm visibly shaking. I can't do this. I'm not yet ready for this bike; it's way out of my league. It's like being handed the keys to a Ferrari right after getting a driver's license. But how am I going to tell Bill and the guys from Cannondale? My parents walk toward me, not saying anything because they saw what just happened. They help me lift the bike back into the SUV and we drive silently back to the bike shop. "That's a great bike," I miserably tell my parents, "but I don't think I'm going to be able to ride it this weekend." They think it's a wise decision.

I inform Bill that I can't ride the Slice. It's too advanced for my skill level. He looks at me and says, "I agree with you 100 percent, but if you finish the race, this bike is all yours. How does that sound?"

I stare at him for several seconds. A weight has been lifted off my shoulders. I give Bill a triumphant high five and tell him that I will do my best on race day.

PEOPLE HAVE ASKED ME WHY I EVEN WANT TO DO THE IRONMAN AFTER going through all that pain and suffering in the recent past. There's an old saying that goes something like this: "A person hasn't lived until he has almost died, and for those who have fought for life, the world has a flavor the protected will never know." Life is all about taking risks and accepting challenges when faced with adversity. This sentiment might seem like a cliché, but to survivors like myself, it means never giving up.

RACE DAY IS HERE. I WAKE UP AT FOUR IN THE MORNING. THE BALCONY outside my hotel room has an ideal view of the Kona pier. There's already plenty of commotion and bright lights. In three hours, I will be swimming in the bay with nearly two thousand other triathletes. I still can't believe it. I sit in the dark in a pair of blue board shorts with a bowl of oatmeal and some coffee, watching and waiting. I finish my breakfast and walk into my parents' room. I can tell by their demeanor that they are more nervous than I am.

As we take the elevator down to the lobby, my mom asks, "Do you think you're really ready for this?"

"Mom, I don't know if I'll finish, but I'm going to give it everything I have."

The elevator doors open and triathletes are moving in every direction, with duffel bags slung over their shoulders and water bottles in their hands. This morning, everyone seems more subdued than usual.

As much as I want to blend in with these serious competitors, I'm hiding behind an artificially confident façade. Deep down, I'm petrified.

We make our way to the pier where I get my race number inked on my arms and legs—163.

I enter the bike transition area—it's a shiny metallic sea of gleaming expensive machinery. It takes me a while to tape all three PowerBars and ten PowerBar gels on top of the handlebars. The other bikes have one or two gels and a single energy bar taped to their top tubes. I feel embarrassed because it looks like I'm getting ready to go on a picnic instead of preparing for a race.

THE COUNTDOWN HAS BEGUN—TWENTY MINUTES TO THE 7:00 A.M. start. I hug my parents and tell them not to worry too much.

I get focused. Really focused.

With my swim cap and goggles dangling in one hand, I walk down the stone steps that lead to the swim start. Because the beach is too small to accommodate all the triathletes, almost everyone self-seeds in the shallow water by swimming out fifty to a hundred yards, with stronger swimmers positioning themselves near the front. That's where I situate myself because I think I can handle it this time. Right in the middle.

The one hundred or so pros take off at 6:45 a.m. with a fifteen-minute head start over the rest of the field. As I tread water waiting for the cannon blast to signal our start, the sun rises over the Big Island mountains to the east.

Then *boom*!

The Ironman begins.

The bay instantly turns into a white chaos of moving bodies. I'm getting kicked, punched, clawed, scratched, dunked, pulled back, and crushed by swimmers, and I'm doing the same right back to them because I learned my lesson the hard way at Steelhead in Lake Michigan. It's dog-eat-dog, every man and woman for themselves. You just have to keep your cool and swim aggressively, which is what I do.

I'm moving along with a steady group of swimmers, but after about twenty minutes, I feel a sharp pain in my right calf. Ah, the most important race of my life and I get a muscle cramp, which is something I've never had before in years of swimming. I try to kick it out by loosening up the tightly clenched muscle fibers. I use my left leg to pick up the slack.

When I reach the halfway point and swim around the stationary boat, I check my watch. Thirty-seven minutes—I'm making good time. I hope I didn't go out too quickly. I have another 1.2 miles to swim.

I ease up a bit heading back to the pier. I swim toward a pack of swimmers and stay behind the feet of a large swimmer. The drafting saves me energy. The pesky leg cramp won't go away, however.

Before long, I approach the pier. I hear the loud roars of spectators cheering and people blowing air horns. As I climb unsteadily up the ramp, an NBC cameraman shadows every step.

I jog through the showers to rinse away the salt water and then pick up my transition bag and change into my bike clothes. I look down at my watch: 1:11. Not bad. I feel rejuvenated. I trot over to where my CAAD8 Cannondale bike awaits and roll it out of the transition area, with the NBC cameraman still trailing closely.

I spot my parents beside the transition exit and give them a thumbs-up as I ride away. The sidewalks are packed with spectators. I feel like I'm riding in the Tour de France. The first few miles of the bike course make a circle around town. Then we climb diagonally up the mountainside on Kuakini Drive south toward a left turn at the Queen K Highway whereupon the road heads north, high above the coast. I'm extra cautious as I follow a long line of cyclists, keeping a safe distance between myself and other riders. I'm holding onto the handlebars for dear life. Several riders have already crashed. Paramedics are carting off one triathlete in an ambulance.

Once I leave town and ride along the Queen Ka'ahumanu Highway, my tension fades because there's a lot more riding room. I'm passed by hundreds of cyclists who cruise right by my left shoulder. I continually hear "on your left" as if it is on a tape loop. I try to pay these other triathletes little heed. But after an hour of pedaling through the bleak lava desert, I'm pretty much riding on my own. I wish there were spectators cheering. Instead, it's just the lonely road, my three bottles of orange Gatorade, a canister of salt pills, two extra tire tubes and a CO_2 cartridge for a flat tire, PowerBar gels and PowerBars—and my random thoughts.

As I'm going up a long sweeping hill, I see a helicopter hovering in the sky up ahead. My goodness! Here come the pros from the other direction. Their speed is awesome. I'm guessing they're biking thirty miles per hour. I wonder what it must be like to be that good.

I'm biking at a steady seventeen- to twenty-miles-per-hour clip. Every fifteen minutes, I take a nice long sip of Gatorade. Every forty-five minutes I eat a PowerBar gel; and every ninety minutes, I have a PowerBar and a salt pill to prevent cramping in the heat. At Steelhead, I barely drank during the bike portion. If I don't stay fed and hydrated in Hawaii, I might as well stand by the side of the road with my thumb out looking for a ride back to the transition area. Some experts say the Ironman isn't simply a race but a marathon eating contest. You can consume up to eight thousand or nine thousand calories in a single day. Nutrition is the fourth discipline in triathlon. I load up with water at the aid stations every ten miles.

About thirty-five miles into the bike portion begins the brutal seventeen-mile climb to the turnaround in the sleepy little village of Hawi. This section of road rises six hundred feet in altitude and often into fierce headwinds. I'm not prepared for this, because I did most of my bike training in a parking lot and around a high school track.

I try to imitate some of the other riders as they labor up the climb. I use the small front chain ring and the largest rear gear cog—the easiest combination. But it takes all my energy to keep my legs pumping. I notice that some riders are not sitting but standing out of their seats. I try that for a while. Adding insult to injury is a howling headwind.

A woman to my left in her late thirties is riding a red Cannondale bike, same model as mine. She's out of her seat pedaling. "Nice bike!" I shout between gasps of air. She looks over with a half smile as sweat rolls down her sunburned face. I can't keep up with her and she pulls ahead.

I suffer in silence, fighting the temptation to stop and rest. Because of the stress from the climb, my right calf seizes up. The cramp from the swim has returned with a vengeance. I'm now primarily pedaling with my left leg, while wiggling my right leg. I'm probably biking at five miles per hour. Any slower, I will fall.

With my body in rebellion, I can no longer postpone the inevitable. I can't go any further. I have to take a break. For how long, I don't know. I click out my left foot from the pedal but right before I come to a complete stop, I'm struck by a powerful mental vision of my parents waiting for me.

Haven't they done enough waiting for me over the years, especially when I was in Intensive Care? For two months, they waited to see if I would wake up, if I would live, if I would be able to speak. Now we have come all this way together, and so why am I questioning whether I have the strength and willpower to bike up this mountain? It's no longer just me doing this race; it's the three of us. This ride to Hawi is a significant piece of the giant puzzle of my recovery. But I can solve it only if I push through the fatigue and pain.

So I don't roll to a stop. I click my left foot back into the pedal, swallow some salt tablets, and continue riding in a renewed frenzy of determination.

I remain in my seat, spinning at a high cadence. When that becomes tiring, I stand on the pedals, mashing them down with exhausted legs. Rivers of sweat are pouring down my face. I feel like I'm riding in an enormous oven and each time my feet rotate, I'm turning up the temperature dial even more.

I'm nearly delirious with suffering. And then, there's salvation, relief from the torment of heat, wind, fatigue. The ascent levels off and Hawi is just ahead. People line the streets, and the cheering provides me with a new source of power and energy. I zip around the turnaround, giving everybody waves and smiles, while preparing myself for the long descent.

The downhill section is terrifying. I'm traveling so fast that the bike begins to shimmy. I must be going at least forty miles per hour. One small mishap and I'll be torn to shreds by the fall. Yet I literally throw caution to the wind. I hold on tighter to the handlebars. It might be called a death grip. But I recognize it as a "life grip." I let out a cry of triumph and victory that acts as an emotional release of all the built-up aggression, bitterness, frustration, and anger from the past few years.

I don't remember the accident on July 6, 2004, so I don't know if my life "flashed before my very eyes" like most survivors say it does, but in this sustained moment, as I'm barreling down the mountain, I start having a series of memory flashbacks: waking up from the coma in the hospital; seeing white-sheet covered dead bodies rolled out on gurneys; having my parents visit three times a day; being confined to a wheelchair. Thoughts are rushing by at such velocity that I can't even keep up with them. When I finally reach the bottom of the mountain, my cheeks are wet—not with sweat but with tears of joy.

Energized and cleansed of emotional pain, I have little difficulty making the fifty-six-mile ride back to Kona. I bike at a steady, moderate pace, with a newfound sense of tranquility and peace. I feel at home on the endless lava fields, with the Pacific Ocean on the right, Kohala mountain to the left, and the tropical sun overhead. This is the happiest day of my life.

After seven and a half hours, I finally arrive at the transition area by the pier. I repeat to myself, "Don't crash now; don't you dare crash!" I cautiously click my feet out of the pedals and a volunteer hurries over to assist me. I have trouble walking, but I have to keep moving if I want to finish before the midnight cutoff. I pick up my run transition bag, then sit down in the changing tent. An NBC cameraman is by my side. Two

Ironman volunteers drape me with cold towels. I'm fumbling to put my running shoes on, as another volunteer dries me off and sprays sunscreen on my sun-baked shoulders.

I stand up on shaky legs and strap a hydration belt around my waist for extra fluids. It's time to go "run" a marathon.

The crowds excite me. I'm drawing energy from all the spectators as I slowly jog through Kona. "Keep it up, number 163! Lookin' good," one lady shouts holding up a big poster board that says Good luck Ironman athletes! When I pass a group of surfer dudes with mohawks who are standing by their sticker-plastered pickups, one yells, "You're a beast!"

A female racer in a sky-blue bikini, sporting an Ironman logo on her gorgeously tanned stomach, smiles at me and says that my running stride looks good. I thank her and do a double take as I pass her.

Even though my legs are stiff and wooden, I make it to the five-mile aid station on Alii Drive in fairly good shape. My sole concern is foot blisters caused by all the cups of water that I've been splashing all over my shoes and socks.

The next several miles become increasingly tough. I decide to walk one minute for every mile jogged. The walking serves as a small reward for making headway.

I begin having tunnel vision, barely noticing any of the other runners, most of whom now pass me. My focus is the hot asphalt and where to place my feet.

My longest training run had been two hours. That took me to ten miles. As I make my way up the steep Palani Road, out of the town, and onto the Queen K Highway, I reach my endurance threshold. Keeping my feet moving is all I can hope for. Right foot, left foot, right foot, left foot, and so on. I have gone from jogging to a light bouncing walk. My pace has slowed to a fifteen-minute mile.

"Hey, Brian! Over here, son, over here." I hear the sound of my dad's voice coming from a large group of people to my left. I see him with my mom. They ask how I'm feeling.

"I'm doing all right. Things are good," I lie with a straight face.

The sun is starting to set on the Queen K. The warm yellows and bright oranges in the sky mix with horizontal bands of blues and purples. The pros and top age-groupers have already finished the race several hours ago. I envy them. I still have a long way to go. At the next aid station, a volunteer hands me a Day-Glo chemical stick to wear around my neck because there are no lights along the pitch-dark Queen K.

I now celebrate each mile with a three-minute walking spree. No matter how badly this hurts, the suffering is only temporary, I keep reminding myself. Nor am I the only one experiencing extreme discomfort. Some runners are bent over like hunchbacks. Others are walking. Several are just standing and trying to rub out a leg cramp. To the few people whom I happen to edge by, I say something motivational, such as "Keep it up," "You're doing good," or "We're almost there." Misery likes company on the Queen K.

Night comes quickly in the tropics. The magical hues and luminescent colors in the sky have faded to black. The solid darkness reminds me of being in the coma. Except for the terrifying dreams, it was absolutely dark most of the time. The only things now visible are neon green glow sticks jiggling about racers' necks.

Unlike other back-of-the-packers, I sometimes have company. Every few minutes, a moped zips past with an NBC cameraman on the back. An NBC red convertible Mustang is also trailing me. Ken the cameraman sits in the backseat. He's a great guy. I met him in September when he came to my house to get footage of my parents and me for the NBC Ironman telecast.

Each mile is devoured in slow motion. Thankfully, it's much cooler. While my body hurts all over from the accumulated exhaustion, it's a different kind of hurt than I experienced in the hospital. Then, the pain was out of my control. I was its unwilling victim. But here, I'm causing the pain by running. It's self-inflicted. I could always stop, quit the race. But that will never happen. I won't allow it.

I finally leave the Queen K and make a left turn onto the road to the Energy Lab. The descent is gentle on my legs. They feel as if they are moving on their own. At the turnaround aid station, music is blasting and volunteers wish me good luck.

The long, gradual climb out of the Energy Lab requires more than luck. I slow to a walk. All of a sudden, I start crying because I realize that I will finish the race.

When I get back to the Queen K, I begin to jog again when a silver Mustang convertible drives up alongside me. It's Bill Rudell and the Cannondale crew who are excited to see that I've made it this far. I have been out on the course for thirteen hours. Only six more miles to the end—little more than ninety minutes if I don't stop.

Another mile later, the three LifeSport coaches pull up alongside me in a car—Lance, Paul, and Alister who have played an important role in my training for the past six weeks and taught me how to do an Ironman virtually overnight. They let me know I'm way ahead of the estimated time they were expecting me to finish—which was close to midnight.

When they leave, Ken and the NBC gang return. It's easy to ignore the all-encompassing exhaustion when a camera is on you.

With just three miles to go, my body will only permit me to walk two hundred yards followed by a painfully slow jog for two hundred yards—walk, slow jog, repeat. My swollen feet feel like cinder blocks and my puffy, swollen legs are barely bending enough to get one foot in front of the other.

I'm so bewildered and depleted by fatigue that I temporarily lose sense of where I am. I have to remind myself that I'm in Hawaii, attempting to finish the Ironman.

With two miles remaining, the NBC camera crew heads back to the finish to await my arrival. I find myself alone in the dark. I savor these last miles, knowing they represent the culmination of a long journey that's taken me from dying to living. When my heart rate was soaring, doctors feared the worse. But now, as my heart is beating strong and fast, I know that I'm living—living my dream.

I make the turn onto Alii Drive. Thousands of spectators line both sides of the street. The finish line is only several hundred yards away. I pick up the pace to an awkward walk and trot. Sheer adrenaline carries me forward.

I see the finish line area, which is lit up like daylight. Fifty yards, twenty-five yards, five yards, then I'm home! I walk across the finish line. My time is fourteen hours and forty-two minutes. An NBC cameraman hovers nearby. My parents rush to greet me. The mood is beyond emotional. Tears. Hugs. Smiles. I feel completely reborn, as if I have been given the gift of a normal life and all the limitations I once had have vanished. Just over three years ago, doctors didn't think I would ever walk again. I had been the boy in the car crash, the dying boy, the boy whose heart stopped numerous times, the coma boy, the boy who couldn't speak or move, the skeleton boy in a wheelchair. But all that is now part of the past on this triumphant night in Kona.

The announcer shouts to the crowd of thousands, "Brian Boyle, at twenty-one years old, is an Ironman!" Yes I am.

EPILOGUE

WHEN I RETURNED HOME FROM HAWAII, A MEDIA WHIRLWIND WAS waiting. I did interviews with local and international newspapers, radio stations, television news programs, and various magazines. But the really big day occurred six weeks later on December 1, 2007, when the ninety-minute Ironman telecast aired on NBC. I watched the show at home with my parents and our bulldog Daisy. It felt great to relive that long day in Kona. Three of the four "inspirational triathletes" finished—Charles Plaskon came in seven minutes after I did, while Scott Rigsby just made the cutoff in 16:42. Sadly, Scott Johnson did not finish. Underlining the greatness of the best professionals were the swift times of the winners: Australian Chris McCormack in 8:15 and Englishwoman Chrissie Wellington in 9:08.

I was flattered to see my personal story highlighted on the NBC show. I thought my fifteen minutes of fame were over, but in the days that followed I was surprised to receive emails from people all over the world. These emails weren't just from fellow auto accident victims, but people who had bouts with cancer, illness, or who had suffered war injuries in

Iraq and Afghanistan. All had experienced life-altering circumstances. All were survivors.

On January 1, 2008, I resumed my triathlon training because I wanted to see if one day I could qualify for the Ironman. With more than six weeks to train this time, I'm giving myself several years to get in the kind of shape I saw in the top triathletes in Kona.

My first step was to sign up for online coaching by six-time Hawaii Ironman champion Mark Allen, who retired from competition in 1996. His personalized training program involves working out anywhere from twenty to thirty hours a week.

Cannondale's Bill Rudell was good with his promise. He sent me the Slice bike as my gift for finishing Kona as well as for being the recipient of the 2007 Cannondale Ironman Determination Award. With the sleek bike, I gradually improved my speed and road-handling skills.

In addition to all the training, I enrolled full-time at St. Mary's. I also continued to get calls from national media reporters. My comeback story appeared on ESPN.com, Comcast Sports, NBC News, Fox News, and in the *Washington Post*. The Catholic monthly *Inside the Vatican* named me as one of its Top Ten People of the Year.

With all this media exposure, I decided to serve as a testimonial speaker with the American Red Cross. Without the thirty-six blood transfusions and thirteen plasma treatments that came from the Red Cross, I never would have made it out of Intensive Care alive. Every two seconds, someone in the United States needs blood. Donors are the only source, so I want to help as much as I can in this vital, life-giving effort.

The next half-Ironman triathlon I did was the Eagleman 70.3 Triathlon in Cambridge, Maryland, on June 8, 2008. I cut two hours off my time from my first race, the Steelhead. Surprisingly, the bike was my strongest of the three disciplines; I was third in my age group.

The next month, I was named PowerBar's Athlete of the Month. I also received the 2008 Fitness Inspiration Award from the IdeaFit World Health and Fitness Association, the ceremony for which took place at the Barry Manilow Theatre in Las Vegas—the same stage where Elvis Presley performed many times. Dan O'Brien, the 1996 U.S. Olympic Decathlon gold medalist, presented me with the award in front of an audience of three thousand.

After returning from Las Vegas, I flew to Canada to compete in the half-Ironman in Newfoundland, where my late grandmother, Helen Lineberger, was raised. I dedicated the race to her memory. The Canadian television news crews, newspapers, and radio stations covered me throughout the entire week. I was able to lower my half-Ironman time another ten minutes.

I was also honored to be included in *Men's Health* magazine's twentieth-year-anniversary edition, which highlighted some of the biggest health and fitness stories over the past two decades. I was awestruck to be included in the same company as Tiger Woods and my personal athletic inspiration, Lance Armstrong.

Right before Christmas, I flew to Clearwater, Florida, to compete in the 2008 Foster Grant Ironman 70.3 World Championship, where I was able to take another twenty minutes off my overall time. It took me only 5:09:14 to finish the race. My grandfather, parents, Aunt Kati, Uncle Tom, and cousins Matt and Hayley, who were always there for me when I was in the hospital and in rehab, came and watched me do the race.

After Florida, I received a call from the *Ellen DeGeneres Show* asking if I would like to be a guest. They wanted to spotlight an Ironman triathlete with an inspirational story. I told the producer I used to watch Ellen's show when I was waking up from my coma and that she was able to make me smile when I was paralyzed.

My parents and I were flown to Los Angeles, California. On the day of the show's taping in the Warner Bros. Studio, I was brought into my own dressing room, which had my name printed outside the door. There was a huge gift basket that included a bathrobe. The two other guests on the show were pop singer Jessica Simpson and actor Chace Crawford, a young star on the popular cable television show *Gossip Girl*. I was the last guest to appear. The lights, camera, and backstage action were overwhelming. Ellen's staff was wonderful. It was incredible to meet Ellen and get the opportunity to tell her how much her show meant to me when I was in Intensive Care.

I haven't slowed down, either. I ran in the March 2009 SunTrust National Marathon in Washington, D.C., and my time was 4:15:12.

While I'm honored by all the media attention and national recognition, it is my intention and desire to make a positive impact on others who have gone through or who are currently going through a tragic, life-altering experience. I was fortunate to be given the gift of life thanks to the support of my parents, hospital, family, and friends. I hope to help other survivors find the faith, confidence, and determination that recovery is within their reach, too.

I still have a lot of ground to cover in life. I will never recapture all that lost time spent in the hospital, or the arduous months of rehab. But that period in my life, I now realize, only marked the beginning of a long unfinished journey. I plan to enjoy every moment.

Life is to be lived. There are no bad days. Every day is a good day.

ACKNOWLEDGMENTS

THIS BOOK IS NOT JUST A STORY OF WHAT I OVERCAME, BUT A STORY of how life can sometimes bring momentous obstacles that need to be conquered, no matter how bleak the situation. Therefore, I must pay tribute to all the following.

The firemen, rescue squads, and helicopter crews who risk their lives everyday to save lives. Much of the time, every second is crucial. These brave men and women are the unsung heroes, and I thank them for getting me out of the car and keeping me alive, both at the scene and in the air:

Accokeek Volunteer Fire Department

La Plata Volunteer Fire Department

Potomac Heights Volunteer Fire Department and Rescue Squad

Tenth District Volunteer Fire Department and Rescue Squad

Charles County Volunteer Rescue Squad

Ironsides Volunteer Rescue Squad

U.S. Park Police Helicopter—Eagle 1

Grateful doesn't even begin to express my deepest appreciation for Prince George's Hospital Center. This facility had the tools to put me back together, and support and encouragement came from the entire hospital—from every area and unit, from the hospital president and the medical departments, to the cafeteria staff, the security, and the parking lot attendants. It became a support system for me and my family. Huge thanks to my physicians, Dr. Said Daee, Dr. James Catevenis, Dr. Mohammad Nafisy, Dr. William Boyce, Dr. Saeed Koolaee, and others for never giving up on me. I'm in awe of what you did for me, and feel that you went above and beyond to save my life. I will be forever grateful as well to my nurses, who cared for me as if I were their son, brother, or even grandson; to Donna Lanier and the radiology department for the endless CAT scans, MRIs and X-rays; to the surgical units that performed the many operations to keep me alive. The expertise, dedication, and teamwork throughout the hospital shone through all my treatment, and I am living proof of their excellence.

I am grateful to Coach Glenn Covey, my high school track coach, for being by my side through the good times and bad. You were even with me in the ICU to cheer me on, but this time you weren't coaching me in a sport but pushing me to fight for my life. I thank you once again.

Appreciation goes to all the blood donors everywhere. Without all of you, I wouldn't be here. I will forever remember your selfless acts of kindness. The American Red Cross blood donor program provides survival to those when least expected.

Working with my good friends, Mike Baisey, Gary Ouellette, and the amazing team at the Greater Chesapeake & Potomac Blood Services Region has been such an honor, and I'm so grateful for all the support that you have shown me over the years. To the President and CEO of the American Red Cross, Mrs. Gail McGovern, thank you for taking the time to write such a sincere and heartfelt introduction to this book; I'm so grateful for all your encouragement and for all that you do for this amazing humanitarian organization.

Kernan Rehabilitation Hospital, thank you for jump-starting my therapy.

My outpatient center, Child and Adult Rehabilitation, provided the intense therapy I needed, and I thank them for working so hard with me and getting my body out of that wheelchair.

To my family, friends, and the supportive people all over the world, thank you for your prayers, letters, cards, and emails with words of encouragement.

I would especially like to thank my cousins, Matt and Hayley, for always standing vigil, literally to my left and right, allowing me to lean on your shoulders during a time when I desperately needed the support or to have a good laugh. You always knew how to put a smile on my face. To my good friends Rachel Gearhart and Jessica Grow for being there throughout my recovery and healing: you both will always have a special place in my heart, more than you'll ever know. To Sam Fleming, thanks for helping me get my swimming back on track, as a coach and as a friend. And, to my grandfather, thank you for always being there for me, in everything that I've done and continue to do in life.

St. Mary's College of Maryland, thank you for your support and encouragement. Thanks especially to my professors: Colby Caldwell, Sue Johnson, Carrie Patterson, Joe Lucchesi, Patrick Kelley, Cristin Cash, Lisa Scheer, David Ellsworth, Ben Click, and Cynthia Koenig. Thanks to Coach Andre Barbins, Assistant Coach Julio Zarate, and my college swim team for making me feel part of the team no matter the outcome.

Thank you, Jay Cutler, for helping me get my muscles back, and Gary Hall, Jr., for your inspiring words, which helped me get back in the pool.

Mahalo to the Hawaii Ironman, World Triathlon Corporation (WTC), NBC, and Peter Henning for allowing me the opportunity to live my life without fear again. My deepest appreciation also extends to these fine people from the WTC: Ben Fertic, Andy Giancola, Blair LaHaye, Bill Potts, Jessica Weidensall, Kevin Mackinnon, Gaylia Lynn Osterlund, and Jennette Harshman. Crossing the finish line in Kona confirmed that my insides were really okay. It was the final healing phase for my body and my spirit. I will always be grateful.

All the sponsors who helped me and continue to support me on my Ironman journey also deserve appreciation and thanks: 4EverFit Nutritional Supplements (which also helped me gain weight back during my rehab), Timex Watches, PowerBar Sports Nutrition, Cannondale Bikes, Profile Design, Foster Grant Sunglasses, Kinesys Sunscreen, Nathan Active Hydration, Newton Running Shoes, and TYR.

Thank you to Skyhorse Publishing and Tony Lyons for believing in this project. I began writing about my journey as another form of therapy in late 2004 after I was released from the hospital. After several years of writing, my literary agent Bill Katovsky, who has been a mentor and editor, helped me realize my dream of getting this book published. Without him, *Iron Heart* (he also came up with the title) would never have happened. He pushed, motivated, and steered me in the right direction through every chapter and almost every sentence of this book. I'm forever grateful for his generosity. Bill taught me how to write from the heart, and that's ultimately the book's foundation.

And, finally, to Mom and Dad: You were there every single day that I was in the hospital. There were only three visiting hours a day, but you got there in the morning and left in the late evening. You were there by my side through the good, the bad, and the horrible. Every time you came in to see me in the hospital, you did not know if I was going to be dead or alive, but you always kept the hope. That hope is what ultimately brought me back from the dead and into life again. Your love saved me, and for that reason, you are my world. Thank you for always believing in me, even when I was too tired and sick to believe in myself. I love you, Mom and Dad. We did it!

AFTERWORD

A LOT HAS HAPPENED IN THE TWO YEARS SINCE IRON HEART WAS FIRST published in hardcover. For the paperback edition I'm happy to bring everyone up to date on what's occurred in my life since then.

This past June, I competed in the Eagleman Ironman70.3 triathlon, a half-Ironman distance race held in Cambridge, Maryland. It was the first time I ever raced in the twenty-five to twenty-nine age group. Out of around 2,500 competitors, I placed eighty-fifth overall with a time of 4:38:13. I not only beat my previous best time by twenty-four minutes, but I also qualified for the Ironman70.3 World Championship in Las Vegas.

Ever since *Iron Heart* came out, it seems that my life is in fast-forward. I have enjoyed the camaraderie of runners at marathons in New York City, Philadelphia, Washington, D.C. and elsewhere. During each of these races, I proudly wore the American Red Cross logo on my racing jersey as a tribute to all the anonymous blood donors whose generosity helped to save my life. I'd often hear spectators or other runners shout, "Go Iron Heart!"

I have continued working closely with the National Headquarters and Greater Chesapeake & Potomac Blood Services Region of the

American Red Cross, showing up at blood drives to offer encouragement to others, giving talks at donor appreciation meetings and hospitals, and working with the students in the Red Cross NAIA Collegiate Leadership Program.

Once, despite several days of severe snowstorms, 1,100 units of blood were collected in a series of blood drives that we arranged. One of the Iron Heart blood drives took place at Prince George's Hospital. To see many of my close friends and relatives come out for the drive and donate was a momentous occasion. But the real highlight was when my heart surgeon, Dr. Naficy, finished up his hospital shift and came in and made his own blood donation. To express my deep appreciation for everyone that played a part in keeping me alive, I was able to make my very first blood donation that same day! Several of the hospital staff teased me by saying that I still owed them thirty-five more pints to make up for what they gave me when I had been a patient.

In 2010, I graduated Cum Laude from St. Mary's College of Maryland. I was also awarded the American Red Cross Regional Spokesperson of the Year award for the second consecutive year. Even though my college degree was in graphic design, my career has increasingly turned to public and corporate speaking. These speaking events take place all across the nation, before various medical organizations, hospital associations, and medical/nursing schools, where I tell my personal story.

Speaking at these medical conferences is a rewarding experience because it allows me the opportunity to show my appreciation for what these healthcare individuals do on a daily basis. As a hospital patient, you are depending on others to help you get through tough, uncertain times as well as support you through various degrees of recovery. Victory is measured in the smallest achievable increments, like blinking, or moving a finger, or standing up and walking. But none of this can be done alone. I know. I have been there.

I have also spent many wonderful, emotionally-charged hours visiting Maryland middle schools and high schools. One event consisted of an essay contest in which students wrote about a time in their life when they encountered a challenging situation. After I shared my story, I had the opportunity to listen to the finalists read their essays to the audience. I was inspired by the experiences of these young students who had to learn firsthand how to deal with a traumatic experience such as their house burning down, taking care of a dying parent or grandparent, defending a friend from a bully, or overcoming an eating disorder. Hearing these young students talk about their own lives made me reflect back to when I was their age and my own life was unexpectedly turned upside down in 2004.

Since this book was first published I've received thousands of emails from people and met hundreds more and everyone had their own story to tell—and I've come to understand that no matter what life throws at you, each of us has the inner strength to overcome these challenges. With the right attitude, we all have the power to move past the hardships and obstacles, while banishing negativity and dark moods to a forgotten place. I truly believe that it is only during your weakest and most vulnerable moments when you find out how strong you really are.

I hope to continue testing myself in difficult athletic endurance events. My sights are set on competing in many more marathons, ultra marathons, and Ironman races. And each time I show up a race, I think about everyone who has helped me succeed along this unexpected path back to the living. Hours later, after crossing the finish line, the joy that I experience is measured not just by how fast I went, but by the joy I feel in living life to the absolute fullest.

Finally, thank you for reading *Iron Heart* and sharing this journey with me. This book opened with me in a hospital room—confused, terrified, immobile, and not knowing where I was. And now, the book closes with me knowing exactly where I am—and where I want to go.

—Brian Boyle,
June 2011, Maryland

ABOUT THE AUTHORS

BRIAN BOYLE's *Iron Heart* blog and contact information can be found at http://brianboyle.wordpress.com.

BILL KATOVSKY is the editor, author, and coauthor of several books, including *Embedded: The Media at War in Iraq*, which won Harvard's Goldsmith Book Prize. A two-time Hawaii Ironman finisher and founder of *Tri-Athlete* magazine, Bill can be reached at katovsky.bill@gmail.com.